Advance Praise for *Chakra Foods for*

"*Chakra Foods* is loaded with wisdom, joy, and practicality. Reading through provided me with many 'ah ha!' experiences. *Chakra Foods* is full of unusual and uplifting insights that one can apply to their life instantly."
—Christiane Northrup, M.D., author of *The Secret Pleasures of Menopause* and *Women's Bodies, Women's Wisdom*

"An original and outstanding work of art and science. Dr. Minich's refreshing approach to energetic and nutritional health reminds us that the food we eat must be viewed with timeless, universal eyes, swallowed with more than just our throats, and assimilated with and into our entire being."
—Kenneth Fine, M.D., founder and director of the Intestinal Health Institute and EnteroLab.com Reference Laboratory

"Anyone looking for a holistic and practical means through which to connect your spirit and well-being to your food must look no further; Minich clearly and simply provides an individualized healing guide to nurture your body's physiology as well as its essence."
—Allison Imel Hamza, nutritional therapy practitioner

"Dr. Minich believes that body and soul are intimately connected to the food we eat. How profound to discover how food nourishes much more than just our bodies. If you are searching for a deeper connection between your body, mind, and spirit, and are striving for a greater sense of contentment, then this is the next on your must-read list! After reading *Chakra Foods for Optimum Health* you will discover what foods will nurture both body and soul and look at food in a deeper, more complex way."
—Barb Schiltz, M.S., R.N., nutritionist

"*Chakra Foods for Optimum Health* shifts the standard diet book paradigm. Instead of offering a superficial or disconnected plan to override unhealthy eating habits, Minich serves a delicious regime of foods and philosophy designed to connect to divine wisdom, inspiration, and joy. Successfully weaving together hard science, ancient spirituality, real life case studies, and mouth watering recipes, *Chakra Foods* couldn't be more innovative or down to earth. Definitely destined to become a classic."
—Elise Marie Collins, author of *Chakra Tonics*

"*Chakra Foods for Optimal Health* is a must-read for anyone seeking to understand their issues around food. Minich creates a nice balance between science and the spiritual. Her left and right brain approach to health is engaging, inspiring, and informative. It will give everyone who reads it lots to 'chew on.'"
—Donna Landry, PAC

"Dr. Minich's book fills a long-time need for a practical approach to food—one that heals and comforts, empowers and emboldens, and invites food to occupy the center of our table in a loving rather than guilt-driven way. This chakra-based method for diagnosing our problems and healing ourselves through food will not only work, but invite brilliance into our lives and world."
—Cyndi Dale, author of *New Chakra Healing* and *The Subtle Body: an Encyclopedia of Your Energetic Anatomy*

"This is a shining work of nourishing wisdom. It carries gifts of clarity for anyone who cares deeply for the soul, body, and mind. And it is a sacred text of action for seeing our bodies as treasures of the living earth."
—Char Sundust, Sundust Oracle Institute

"For years, Americans have had a serious love/hate relationship with food which focuses on avoidance and guilt. *Chakra Foods* artfully guides the reader away from the path of love/hate to a place of love/love. . . . [The] consumption of fast foods is slowly becoming a thing of the past. *Chakra Foods for Optimum Health* is a dietary door to the future."
—Adam Banning, lecturer, radio personality, functional medicine consultant, and author of *Seeing the Angel in the Mirror*

"In this monumental work, Minich has uniquely intertwined the power of our everyday interaction with food to the interconnected dynamic of our intuitive energetic key that locks or unlocks our ability to heal. She . . . guides you through the information in a way that is like nothing else you have experienced. This work will be beneficial for patients and professional medical practitioners alike."
—Barbara Maddoux, R.N., D.O.M.

"*Chakra Foods for Optimum Health* is a 'roll up your sleeve' self-help book. Filled with 'that's me!' case histories, it skillfully weaves science, physiology, psychology, energy medicine, and ancient medical wisdom into an accessible framework that will help you chart your journey back to health, creativity, and love.

It is beautifully and poetically written and will resonate with your mind, your heart, and your soul."
—Jacob Kornberg, M.D., F.A.C.S.

CHAKRA FOODS

for

Optimum Health

A GUIDE *to the* FOODS
that can IMPROVE YOUR ENERGY, INSPIRE
CREATIVE CHANGES,
OPEN YOUR HEART, *and*
HEAL BODY, MIND, *and* SPIRIT

Deanna M. Minich, Ph.D., C.N.

Conari Press

First published in 2009 by Conari Press,
an imprint of Red Wheel/Weiser, ᴏꜰ
With offices at:
500 Third Street, Suite 230
San Francisco, CA 94107
www.redwheelweiser.com

ISBN: 978-1-57324-373-5
Library of Congress Cataloging-in-Publication Data
Minich, Deanna.
  Chakra foods for optimum health : a guide to the foods that can improve
your energy, inspire creative changes, open your heart, and heal body, mind,
and spirit / Deanna Minich.
      p. cm.
  Includes bibliographical references and index.
  ISBN 978-1-57324-373-5 (alk. paper)
  1. Chakras. 2. Food--Miscellanea. I. Title.
  BF1442.C53M56 2009
  613.2--dc22
                          2008041150

Cover design by Maxine Ressler
Text design by Donna Linden
Typeset in Perpetua, Priori Sans, and RuseX000HG
Cover photographs: Water © David Joyner/iStockphoto.com, Blackberries © Elena Asenova/ iStockphoto.com, Kiwi © Drew Hadley/iStockphoto.com, Avocado © Raychel Deppe/ iStockphoto.com, Corn © Sandra Caldwell/iStockphoto.com, Orange © Klaudia Steiner/ iStockphoto.com, Red onion © Massimiliano Pieraccini
Interior illustration, page 16 © Song Speckles/iStockphoto.com

Printed in the United States of America
IBT

To Sharon——my mother, teacher, and friend,
who led me to this rainbowed path

CONTENTS

ACKNOWLEDGMENTS

Giving thanks is one of the best parts of writing a book. You don't do anything alone in life, and it's so rewarding to step back and admire the web you are intimately enmeshed in. Writing these acknowledgments gives me this opportunity.

Above all, my deepest, most soul-full, heart-full gratitude goes to Spirit . . . for the inspiration, knowledge, and seamless thread of words that were gifted to me and flowed from my fingers to the keyboard.

I often tell others that I wouldn't be speaking or writing about this material if it weren't for my mother. Not just because she gave birth to me, but also because her epiphany when I was nine years old fueled so much of what my life is about now: food and spirituality. I admire her grace, strength, and dedication to her true path. She set an example for me to live my life to the fullest. I am grateful to the rest of my family: Dad, for instilling the genes of passion within me; Brenda, for her sharp-mindedness and humor; and Ian, for his bountiful creativity.

My (spiritual) teachers, Patrice Connelly, Cyndi Dale, Char Sundust, Caroline Myss, Louise Hay, Jeffrey Bland, and Paramahansa Yogananda, have imparted gracious gifts of wisdom, insight, and love—all of which have made a profound difference in my life.

I give heartfelt thanks to all of the participants who took part in *Nutrition for the Soul* classes and workshops, especially those who helped me get them started in the summer of 2007. Without all of your continuing requests for this book, I may not have had the same drive to get this material into book form. Therefore, I write this for all of you. You've helped me to implement what I was inspired to create.

My heart extends those who have helped me in the publishing process: my agent, Krista Goering, for passionately believing in this text and being able to take it to the next level, and my remarkable editor at Red Wheel, Caroline Pincus.

And finally . . . I bow to my teacher, my support, my love . . . Mark.

PREFACE

Perhaps you've been working on small pieces of yourself—like your diet, or becoming more aware of your body, or maybe you've been exploring your spirituality. I have noticed that many people are hungry for a spiritual connection with something greater than themselves. Their souls wander a path of longing and questioning. Similarly, others struggle with the needs of their physical bodies. They are in continual search for the ultimate understanding of why they remain unsatisfied with their appearance or why they have numbing pain. Still others are confused about how to eat. Their minds are swirling in all the diet information that bombards us on a daily basis. And most of us, if presented with the choice, would want to have it all: how to bring our bodies and souls to a higher, more contented spot and park there indefinitely.

Of course, we cannot live without the body or the soul, as both are wrapped into one—it's a package deal. As you will read in the following pages, nutrition, body, and spirituality form a solid, inseparable triangular relationship. The mission of this book is to help you understand your relationship to food and eating so that you may bridge together body and soul, to be and feel complete, whole, and full of love. Of course, food and eating present powerful options to unite body and soul; however, keep in mind that they represent one path into the whole of your being. To fully support your growth and evolution, it is also essential to shift not only your eating, but your whole way of life, including your thoughts, actions, activities, and beliefs. Changing your eating is an important step in that process.

To help you arrive at the "sweet spot" of unifying all aspects of the self using the conduit of food, I have blended a dash of science and generous amounts of intuition and training into a foundation of spirituality. The spiritual template I use is one based on the ancient system of chakras established by East Indian yogis, which is cultivated through the art of yoga and threaded through timeless Vedic texts.

Choosing the chakras to combine with foods and eating became an obvious choice to me as a nutritionist who practices yoga and has studied the chakras through books and experientially. And, most of all, it worked! I noticed in my consultations with individuals that many imbalances in the chakras coincided with food issues. For example, several people with solar plexus chakra deficiency, who felt stressed and worn out by their environment, also revealed to me that they had issues with sugar. Indeed, I discovered with my blended intuitive and physiological perspectives that these two seemingly disparate presenting complaints were actually interrelated and woven into each other. The nutritional advice I was accustomed to giving individuals extended not to only food advice but also tips on living life in a balanced way for that particular chakra. Each instructional piece strengthened the other.

When I tell many people about the relationship between chakras and foods, they understand immediately. It's a logical fit. After all, chakras are energy centers in the entire being, and food provides energy to feed these aspects of ourselves. *Chakra Foods* gently walks you through the journey of your energetic landscape and gives you creative tools and insight as to how foods and ways you eat can heal, brighten, balance, and strengthen parts of you that need not only physical, but spiritual nourishment. Every chapter of *Chakra Foods* dives into a single chakra, its physical correlates, and all of its energetic intricacies that manifest in our lives as emotional tumult or physical breakdown. With this information, you will be equipped to create a healing path to this part of yourself, with specific foods resonant with that chakra and even ways to eat to tune into that chakra.

There is no one diet that will work for an entire population of people. That would be too easy. We are all so incredibly unique from a biochemical perspective. Our multifaceted chakra network provides an additional overlay of complexity that interacts with our diverse biology. Therefore, we shortchange ourselves when we stuff our beautiful diversity and complexity into a stifling, static "diet," or path. It is like wearing a dress that does not fit. It is uncomfortable, looks terrible, and we just want out! No "one" ultimate solution exists. If we could piece apart the body and soul aspects of ourselves and deal with the parts of our being as if they were in silos, our lives might be radically different. However, we are a uniform whole; all of the aspects of our being are equally important and must be recognized.

For optimal wellness, the gap between our earthly body and ethereal soul must be closed, integrating throughout in harmony. We evolve over the course of our lifetimes, dealing with different emotional states and situations, all intricately interplaying with our physiology, making us need different foods at specific times. Even Buddha was said to have been worn out from a diet of root vegetables over an extended period of time. No one food (or diet) fits one soul or one body. We must be continually in tune with our changing and cascading needs. *Chakra Foods* opens up the doorway to making sense of the complexity of who you are, being able to "read" this complexity through your eating patterns and through the chakra imprints.

Why food? The one premise that I believe most professionals and laypeople would agree upon and that has remained consistent is that food has an amazingly potent effect on the emotions, body, mind, and spirit, and, conversely, our food choices affect these parts of us as well. By hitting the internal "reset button" to arrive at our inherent, intuitive baseline, we can eat in harmony with who we are as unified body and soul. When we function as an optimally resonating collective, we can be grounded and creative in the present moment. We can focus on tasks at hand, helping us to feel a sense of accomplishment. We are able to take better care of ourselves when we know what we need moment to moment. Therefore, we will have more radiant bodies—we will be our perfect weight, shine forth our radiance through clear eyes and skin, speak our truth without the layering of lies and deceit to others and ourselves, harness a wealth of energy so we are not dragging throughout our days, and be able to connect creatively with elements at hand to tap into the universe of opportunities available to us at all times.

One of the ways to come to this place of balance is to get in touch with the soul needs; this can be done through working with the chakra system. Foods can take us to the realm of heightened energy, glowing health, and vibrancy by feeding the energetic layers of the chakras.

The food-spirit connection is what *Chakra Foods* is about. It takes you to the other side of the spectrum by giving you the tools to fuse the connection between body and soul through the physical and vibratory qualities of food and in how we approach foods and eating.

I am grateful to be able to provide you with this approach to add to your palette of choices for achieving wellness. For some of you, it may simply be a stepping-stone on your way to your truth; and for others, it may change your life dramatically. Either way, I wish you the simple, perfect, shining health we are endowed with and always have access to, and must find again if we are feeling lost.

Deanna M. Minich, Ph.D., C.N.
Port Orchard, Washington
Summer 2008

MY RAINBOWED BEING

I am red.
Passionate, warm, connected to the roots of earth.
An eclipsed sun blessing a sacred union—
A tapestry of soul created from the threads of ancestors.
Pure acceptance of the self, breathing in trust, living to the beat of the heart.
Tiptoeing into the mystery.

I am orange.
Overflowing with expression, bursting forth with raw creation.
Swimming in the depth of feelings—
Juicy bites of life fill the belly with sweetness.
Creatures of land, air, and water unite.
The spiraling energy of the whirling Dervish—
an endless dance of giving and receiving and sharing!

I am yellow.
Illuminating brilliance, power, and intellect.
An exploding bouquet of flowers, an infinite buffet of food and drink—
The exuberance of the sun, the wisdom of Saturn
Embracing with its warmth, marching to the rhythm of life.
It is shiny gold, worth more than any currency.

I am green.
A lotus flower in full-bloom residing in the lushness of the heart.
Reaching, embracing, nourishing all in need.
Fragile as the morning dew, as expansive as the depth of fragrant forests.
Ultimate unconditional acceptance,
like the Mother Earth's love for her children.

I am blue.
Calm and cool, a reflection in a mirrored pond.
Diamond stars married to the nighttime sky.
The ocean waves curling back to their source.
Kind, compassionate words serving as our guide, teacher, and mentor.
Father Sky carries truth in the celestial music of his voice.

I am purple.
The richness of velvet and the elegance of silk.
Diamonds of intuition embedded in the space of all-knowingness.
Imagination running through the vastness of the dreamscape,
playing in a field of swaying lavender, swirling in the energy of dimensions.
Insight radiates softly into the mind's eye.

I am white.
Living within us like the innocence of a child.
Sitting quietly, still with peace and patience, ready to serve.
Every sparkling, dazzling particle on our planet shining forth universal light.
The phenomenal beauty of pure Spirit.

I am many colors.

NOTE TO READERS

This book is intended as an informational guide and is not meant to treat, diagnose, or prescribe. For any medical condition, physical conditions, or symptoms, always consult with a qualified physician or appropriate health care professional. Neither the author nor the publisher accepts any responsibility for your health or how you choose to use the information contained in this book.

Names and identifying details have also been changed to honor people's desire for confidentiality.

CHAPTER I

THE VIBRATION OF FOOD
AND THE SPIRIT OF EATING

We are indeed much more than what we eat, but what we eat
can nevertheless help us to be much more than what we are.
—ADELLE DAVIS

WE ARE "ONIONED" BEINGS

If you are reading this book, chances are you understand that a human being represents the whole of several compressed layers, similar to those of an onion. Healing can occur by peeling away the layers. When we reach one layer, such as the emotional layer, and make a change, no matter how small or big, it ripples into every other aspect of our being like a droplet of water losing itself into a pond. For seconds afterward, the pond is filled with the rhythmic beauty of concentric circles. The pond has been changed forever because of that single, innocent droplet.

Knowing that anything we do to ourselves affects our energetic fabric and, in turn, our physical bodies implies that we can choose to focus on any means of healing that attracts us in order to help heal ourselves. Food and nutrition are avenues that some people choose as paths to their physical and spiritual healing. If you are especially drawn to diets and nutrition, it may simply be that food is your conduit of healing—the medium upon which you learn your life lessons, temporarily or for the extent of your Earth journey.

No matter the path choice, the vehicle will be symbolic in diverse ways. Every path we choose will have intention and be laden with messages if we allow ourselves to receive them. An underlying principle to remember throughout this book, and any book you read on food and eating is that *our relationship to food and eating is symbolic of how we approach everything else in our lives.* Do you eat convenience foods because you are always on the run? Perhaps you need to look at what you are running from—where does your focus need to be, or what do you need to make time for? Or are you eating alone, secretly, especially if you are feeling emotional? If so, what needs to come out in the open? What needs expressing? Who do you need to surround yourself with?

> Our relationship to food and eating is symbolic of how we approach everything else in our lives.

Certainly, our relationship to food can open us up to insight about what our lives are like. It has been said that "As within, so without"—our internal environment mirrors our external surroundings. Our restoration to wellness lies in our awareness of what envelops us, how we engage with the world—with food and eating. The impact that food choices can have on our health can be significant, especially due to the sheer quantity of food we eat throughout our lifetimes—estimated to be at 60,000 to 100,000 pounds—and the fact that we *need* food to exist on this planet.

In fact, we are given many opportunities to make food selections that benefit the layers of our complex selves. A modest calculation of three meals a day, 365 days a year, for an average life span of seventy-six years would mean that we have nearly 84,000 opportunities to have meaningful, healing interactions with food! There is unleashed potential in every single interface with food: each exchange carries the ability to bring you to a higher state of health, to keep you where you are currently at, or to take you into a state of symptoms or add to the pending avalanche of symptoms culminating in disease. Therefore, I encourage people to ask their bodies before making a food selection as to whether the food(s) will help or hurt them.

In the grand theater of life, food has the center stage, as it serves our most primal need for survival, our bond with the Earth, and our intimate connection with each other. We link ourselves to all living beings on the planet through the process of eating and being a participant in the food chain. As a result, our incessant interaction with food takes on immense power and can define who we are. It is no wonder that people have strong opinions about how to eat.

Despite being continually surrounded by food in all forms, ranging from 24-hour grocery stores to deluxe drive-thrus to vending machines, its existence and our innate need for it are ironically ignored. In the whirlwind of busy days, how many of us have thought to ourselves, or expressed to others, that having to eat gets in the way of doing more important things? Some people admit that they simply "forget" to eat. How can we neglect something as crucial for our survival—what message is this sending forth? When we finally do make time to eat, we find ourselves unable to stop due to an unconscious longing for greater satisfaction and union in the midst of our short, sound-bite-laden society and frequent, fleeting social interactions with others. However, with each hurried, unconscious bite, we step further away from merging with everything that food connects us to: ourselves, community, and the Divine. These surface observations indicate that our umbilical relationship with food has been severed, resulting in the fragmentation of the many aspects of ourselves.

Three meals a day, 365 days a year, for an average life span of seventy-six years would mean that we have nearly 84,000 opportunities to have meaningful, healing interactions with food!

Rather than experience a deeper level of understanding about the foods our bodies need for growth and maintenance, people in search of a solution fixate on the path of least resistance, or short-term, quick-fix tools. Is it any wonder that the "diet" approach to eating is a roller coaster of disappointment? Actually, the answers we are so earnestly craving lie before us: at the dining room table, at the restaurant, at the grocery store, and in the garden. Within the eating experiences are planted the true root of what needs healing at our innermost core. When we pay attention to what our body requires and view foods as healing entities, we get right to the heart of why we have manifested chronic diseases or eating dysfunctions. By envisioning foods as dancing molecules of energy that have power and potential to uncover our highest selves, we make food choices to support life-giving thoughts, feelings, beliefs, and actions. Lives can be revolutionized completely by altering our view of food! And the beauty of this miracle is that it can start as soon as your next bite. . . .

Fortunately, our quick-fix eating habits have started to unravel. For example, the "slow food" movement, which encourages the longer, savory experience of eating a gradually cooked meal at a restaurant, has emerged as the antithesis to fast food. Local, organically grown foods and free-range, animal-sourced foods are a prevalent new trend, perhaps even the "hip" way to eat by younger generations. We are gradually returning to a very simple yet profound interaction with food.

FOOD BEYOND THE CALORIE

Although there is much recent news about food being capable of affecting us on many levels (physical, emotional, mental, and spiritual), this realization was brought to light thousands of years ago by ancient traditions like East Indian Ayurvedic medicine and traditional Chinese medicine. In both these traditions, balancing the energetic properties of different foods in the diet is strongly emphasized. For example, in Chinese medicine, foods are selected according to their warming, cooling, drying, or moistening effects on the body. To the novice, it would be relatively easy to intuitively select foods that embody certain properties, as the principles parallel the concepts found in nature. For instance, in general, "warming" foods are those that rev metabolism and create heat in the body. Curried chicken is a good example of a warming food, as it is an animal product and includes seasoning. Both features make the chicken a "hot" food, and it is usually recommended that individuals with a "warm nature" or who are prone to overheating moderate their consumption of these foods. On the other hand, cooling foods would be those that are more neutral in taste and tend not to be cooked, like sliced cucumber or tofu. In contrast to warming foods, they dampen the metabolism, slowing it down. Current Western medicine does not promote the use of foods to prevent disease as much as these other cultures do; however, this trend is changing with new "functional medicine" or "integrative (holistic) medicine," which honors the inner communication between body systems and focuses on the individual as a whole.

Overall, the field of nutrition as a science has been very physically grounded in the basic elements of physiology—such as ingestion, digestion, absorption, transportation, utilization, and excretion of food substances—and the effect of these processes on health. Although physical aspects of food are emphasized in the nutritional paradigm, there is increasing research in the area of the emotional effects of eating. The remaining missing piece is the integration of our body needs with those of our soul and using the needs of one to heal the other. Some may suggest that many people in Western society are not in touch with their soul. It has been said that "illness is the Western form of meditation"— that we do not engage deeper, soulful parts of ourselves unless we are catastrophically provoked. Since chakras span the body and nonbody (soul) parts of our being, they are an excellent way to access the body-soul connection. By tapping into what our chakras are telling us, we are able to better make choices that support integration of our layers of being.

Understanding our health through our chakras enables us to move beyond ensuring that the body has physical food for energy to live by taking us into the realm of food as "spiritual sustenance" or "food for the soul." The synergy of chakras and food provides a superhighway to accessing spirituality, or our interconnectedness with all of life. Together, the chakras and food help us to recognize that life is greater than the sum of its parts. When we shed the idea of food being functional and replace it with choosing to eat to feel the gentle weblike connection with all of life, food takes on a note of Divinity and sacredness. Many cultures and religions have created spiritual practices—such as giving thanks ("grace") for the meal—around eating as a way of acknowledging this sacred act.

> Understanding our health through our chakras enables us to move beyond ensuring that the body has physical food for energy to live by taking us into the realm of food as "spiritual sustenance" or "food for the soul."

UNLOCKING THE SECRET MESSAGES OF FOODS

Emerging science is shedding light on perhaps another dimension to the already existing nutrition foundation. In addition to providing energy, or calories, for the body to function, constituents within food act as messengers that communicate with our body's DNA and influence, to a large extent, the types of proteins and other compounds that cells manufacture. Taking this a step deeper, into the atomic level, the vibrating energetic charged particles of food interact to a significant degree electrically within the fluid matrix inside the body. These vibrations ripple through the system, creating a surge of electrical currents to enhance or deplete the energy state of the cells. The takeaway is that food carries information that will signal our bodies to create proteins to support a vital, creative, optimal structure or to lead to dysfunctional states such as inflammation and pain.

Colorful foods

"Rainbowed eating" is one of the keys to enhancing the whole of our selves.

Nutritionists are taught in school that proteins and carbohydrates both create the same energy currency within the body. For every gram of protein or carbohydrate eaten, 4 kilocalories of energy are available to use. It is now known that these basic nutrients, despite the fact that they are similar in calories, have a different vibration or electrical potential. People can consume the same number of calories, but the metabolic effects within the cells can be different. Protein from vegetables like soybeans and protein from animals like milk-derived casein create different responses in the body even though both are protein. Therefore, the new message is that the *quality* of food, and the dietary signature it carries for the cells, is perhaps most essential.

Unfortunately, it appears that the American profile of eating, referred to by some as the Standard American Diet (S.A.D.), has a deficit of good food signals. We are eating what I like to call the "Brown, Yellow, and White Foods Diet" because it is limited in supplying us with abundant, healthy compounds from plants ("phytochemicals") that equip our cells to work optimally. The food industry has stripped away the colors of foods to give us processed cereals, breads, meats, flours, and baked goods. We are left with lackluster eating, devoid of the rich, flavorful phytochemicals that send high-quality information to our cells, allowing us to flourish. Each compound of color, whether the purple anthocyanidins found in grapes or the red lycopene in tomatoes, has a specific function in the body. If we omit a color from the rainbow spectrum, we are not providing ourselves with the physiological and spiritual functions of that vibration. Hence, as you will uncover in subsequent chapters, "rainbowed eating" is one of the keys to enhancing the whole of our selves.

Not only is the quality of food important, but also *how* the food is eaten. Think of all the health benefits of the Mediterranean diet. Do you think this region of Europe experiences less cardiovascular complications because they eat whole foods rich in precious plant compounds that are heart-protective and antiaging? Most likely, but perhaps not entirely. One point that is often overlooked is the manner in which Mediterranean natives eat: a meal is an event potentially lasting for hours in the company of friends and family. Eating in these countries is an important social event, and working hours are adjusted to accommodate longer lunches, enabling the individual to go home to eat and relax before returning to work again. Imagine how little stress is felt when you have 2 hours to eat lunch versus 30 minutes, and how that can impact your physiological and spiritual responses to food! Eating under pressure may result in absorbing fewer nutrients and feeling ungrounded.

> Without a sense of pleasure and being present in the moment of eating, we may want to eat more to satisfy our need to connect with the experience.

Eating begins before and lasts after the first bite is taken. It starts in the grocery store when we are engaged in food selection or as far back as the field when we planted seeds in the soil. In the grocery store, what colors call out to us? What shapes, forms, tactile sensations, words on packages invite us to buy them? How mindful are we when we grocery shop, or are we distracted by cell phone calls or mental preoccupation with the day's events? If we are growing our own food, are we conscious of the quality of soil we use, our mindset when we are watering the plants, the location in which the seeds are planted? The process of eating continues to the stage of meal preparation, where we gift our olfactory sense with rich aromas and heightened flavors, eventually signaling our gastric juices to begin flowing and specific gut peptides for satiety to be released. If we make a meal with others, in a community setting, the quality of the experience expands many times, as it magnifies our interconnection with others. After the meal, the eating experience continues on the physiological level through the processes of digestion, absorption, and assimilation. If we eat quickly, without mindfulness, we may not be efficient at integrating these food messages into our body and soul. Without a sense of pleasure and being present in the moment of eating, we may want to eat more to satisfy our need to connect with the experience. Therefore, eating while doing other things, such as driving in a car, watching TV, or reading a book, may take away healing energy from the eating experience rather than provide it.

QUANTUM "PHOODS"

Indeed, modern physics gives a whole new twist on how to view living matter. Essentially, all living organisms are compositions of cosmic, dynamic, responsive particles vibrating at a specific frequency. It has been said that the building block of life, the atom, is made of more than 90 percent empty space, implying that only about 10 percent of what is seen as the organism is actual reality. The chunk of most physical life-forms is vibrating energy. These particles of dancing matter form a web of connection, sending signals and creating patterns, vortices, and cascading effects. Therefore, when we think of ourselves as molecules in motion, it is highly plausible that the frequency generated by these interacting particles is modified by our thoughts, our words, the air we breathe, and even the food we eat. In support of this concept, many published research studies, such as those on meditation, prayer, visualization, and diet, support that our minds, words, and environment are powerful and, in ways beyond our understanding, influence emotional, mental, and physical makeup.

We are energy. Animals are energy. Plants are energy. Water is energy. Air is energy. It follows that foods created from animals and plants are energy. Just as each human being is multidimensional and complex, with layers upon layers of emotions, thoughts, history, and potential, so is each living organism. Each animal or plant is composed of the same fine vibrating matter, and like humans, some vibrate quickly and some more slowly. The vibration of food interacts with our inherent vibration, and an exchange of energy occurs. When we feel stuck in a way of thinking or move slowly through the day, eating beef, which carries slower vibrations, adds to our feelings of lethargy. However, when we eat a spicy black bean dish, with spices and beans carrying a higher resonance of energy than that of beef, we stay alert and energetic for hours after eating.

The fact that foods have vibrations is not new. The *Bhagavad Gita* classifies foods containing a relatively high energy vibration or promoting purity and vitality of body and soul as *sattvic*. They are not expensive for the body to process, and they do not leave behind harmful toxins. These foods are described as "savory, smooth, firm, and pleasant to the stomach" and are in contrast to foods that are *rajasic* or "excessively pungent, sour, salty, hot, harsh, astringent, and burnt" and lead to sickness. Examples of sattvic foods include those that are mild, cooling, and refreshing, such as fruits, vegetables, raw milk, clarified butter (known as *ghee*), and honey. Meats are perceived as rajasic, as the flesh is thought to harbor the fear and anger of the animal being killed, transferring it to the eater.

In modern society, there are foods considered to be toxic to our life energy. These foods have been damaged through processing, such as overcooking, burning, mechanical overprocessing, and oxidizing. Recent scientific studies have shown that foods that have been browned through cooking—such as the crust of bread or the brown color of baked products like waffles—age and inflame our cells. (When a protein and a carbohydrate are in the presence of heat, they form a compound that results in a brown color, known as a "Maillard reaction.") Acrylamide and rancid fats are examples of toxic compounds that form in products like potato chips when the potato slices are heated in oil. Therefore, the manner in which food is prepared determines its vibration and its contribution to our energy. Meals made up of leftovers may seem convenient; however, many times they are devoid of any life-giving energy. Rather than give energy, they deplete energy.

> The vibration of food interacts with our inherent vibration, and an exchange of energy occurs.

Food imparts its own healing vibrational energy, and it is responsive to external attitudes, thoughts, words, and actions, regardless of whether from plant or animal, or quick or slow vibration. In other words, we add to the vibration of foods through our thoughts, intentionally bumping up or eroding the healing transformation potential that is part of the food. By putting energy into food, we interact much more deeply with it during eating. If we put positive energy into it and have good thoughts while eating, the food transmits an exponential increase of positive energy in the eating process. On the other hand, if we are hurried, angry, or upset, these feelings transmit through foods into the body, down to the cellular level. Japanese researcher Masaru Emoto, Ph.D., demonstrated this idea best in his book, *The True Power of Water*. Although he is most recognized for his work on the responsiveness of water crystals to words, he did a series of experiments with cooked white rice. He put the cooked rice into two separate jars, one with a taped-on label with the Japanese characters for "You fool" and the other with a label of "Thank you." Over time, the rice inside the jar labeled "You fool" turned black with decay while the rice labeled "Thank you" became yellow because of a lesser degree of degradation. Simply put, words carry energy and affect the vibration of food, causing it to take on that energy. Hence, even *written* words influence the energy of foods.

EATING WITH CONSCIOUSNESS

The way to getting the most out of our food is to be fully present when we are in *its* presence. In fact, this point could be even more essential than the food itself. Our thoughts and beliefs are readily infused into foods and beverages. Although the energy the food brings is important, more important is the energy we bring into the process of eating it and experience from it in our interchange. Our consciousness with food begins with the moment we are choosing it, whether it is at the grocery store, farmer's market, or restaurant. It involves appreciating and giving gratitude to every step involved in that product and thereby honoring its sacredness. The act of eating food is sacred because it can draw us into the cosmic unification we have with all of nature. The gratitude we express for a plant or animal giving up their energy for the sake of our energy is interwoven with our evolution as conscious beings. When we chew our food, it is imperative that we are present in that experience, knowing that we are participating in the process of transformation of energy. Each bite captures the entire energy of the food, from a physiological breakdown to raw energy for use by the cells. All the way back to the energies of the people involved in growing it, manufacturing or harvesting it, choosing and preparing it, every morsel contains an energetic lineage that we can tap into if we are fully present in the moment during our interaction and exchange with food.

With the idea of conscious eating comes the inevitable question of whether we can appreciate processed food like shelf-stable, premade products the same way we can unprocessed, whole foods, and my short answer is *Yes*. With the processed food in mind, we would simply give thanks and recognition to all the individuals involved in its manufacturing. For something like a processed ready-to-eat cereal, we might think about the fields of grain it came from, the people working in the fields selecting and harvesting the grain, the individuals who took care in transporting the grain, the product developers who created the product, and the people wielding the creative genius to put all the ingredients together for a final product. Each step along the way can be filled with gratitude and love for those involved, including the plant or animal food in its whole form. Of course, I am not justifying the consumption of nutrient-poor, highly refined products, but I recognize that the physical and spiritual properties of foods can be transformed through our thoughts and feelings about them.

CHAPTER 2

OUR DANCING CHAKRAS

Everything in the universe has rhythm. Everything dances.
—MAYA ANGELOU

WE ARE MORE THAN OUR PHYSICAL BODIES

The twenty-first century is a time like no other, because science and technology are at an all-time peak. As a society, we have become smitten with all the gadgets, electronics, and high-speed communication potential available, and if we are not conscious of technology's impact, we risk becoming slaves to its appeal.

Your daily events might resemble something similar to the following: waking up to the beeping of an alarm clock, exercising on an automated treadmill while watching the news on the latest flat-screen television, followed by driving to work in your hybrid vehicle while talking on the cell phone, and spending most of the day at work glued to the computer answering emails and plugging in appointments on your Palm Pilot. When it comes to health care, technology may expand its reach by having your medical care be determined by your unique genetic code. Imagine the scenario of going to your doctor with a CD-ROM that contains the contents of your DNA so that your body's code can be read and analyzed instead of talking with a practitioner who observes your symptoms. There is no doubt about it: we are enrobed by technology and tickled by the possibilities it may bring forth.

On the opposite end of the spectrum, we are also becoming more open to the possibility that life provides us more than cold, sleek machines and numbers. Inherently, you may feel and even be reminded through your life experiences that we are more than our physical bodies, and that the human being machine is the best design available. Even though technology gives us the option to connect faster and better, there is truly no replacement for the in-flesh human interaction. The New Age movement, which roughly began in parallel with the proliferation of scientific developments, recognized these ideas and brought them forth as new concepts founded, in part, on ancient, traditional knowledge. If you have experienced Reiki, hands-on healing, prayer, flower essences, homeopathic remedies, herbs, acupuncture, cranial sacral therapy, to name a few, then you have already taken part in the search to heal yourself from a different entry point than modern medicine offers. Not everyone responds in the same way to the same modality, which is why it is so valuable to have a smorgasbord of options available. The current trend is to work with a "healing team" of individuals so that they can use many different approaches to heal.

The nature of science is to understand the body through slicing, dicing, and teasing apart the complexities and intricacies of the human body. Of course, this is valuable to a certain extent, as it allows you to dive down as deep as the gene level to see what you have been programmed with. On the other hand, philosophical, religious, and spiritual teachings promote the wholeness of the person (including the soul) rather than piecing apart our contents into their minutia. As a result, these two paradigms have unique positions that allow them to come together to unlock the mystery of our being. The richness of human healing may be the place where these two paths intersect.

The chakras are the basic foundation of our soul, connecting it to all layers of our being, including our physical body.

Although seemingly disconnected ways of thinking, the two streams of science and spirituality have revealed to us a common thread: that we are essentially compositions of cosmic, dynamic, responsive particles vibrating at a specific frequency. These particles of dancing matter form a web of connection with each other, sending signals and creating patterns, vortices, and cascading effects. One of the ways to tap into our soul selves involves a merging of the physical, emotional, mental, and spiritual by accessing our vibrational selves. Many authors and researchers have begun to explain what that means.

The idea that we are more than our physical body is not a new concept. Traditional spirituality and philosophy, as originated in India and other parts of Asia thousands of years ago, have supported the idea that we are *more* than our physical bodies. Underlying the physical body are other less visible layers, lacing us with the energetic framework for the body template. This layer of our being is fueled by the universal life force that runs through us like electricity, referred to by some as *chi, prana,* or *Divine light,* a concept threaded throughout all major spiritual traditions. Ancient traditions teach that the core of this energy is present in the spinal column, running from the top of the head to the bottom of the spine. From the medical perspective, we could say that this energetic super-highway is analogous to the central nervous system, residing in the spine with distinct clusters and branches that extend throughout the body's surface area.

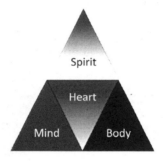

CHAKRAS ARE ENERGY CENTERS

All life-forms, including human beings, have inherent energy vibrations culminating from the cell's electrical activity. Basic biology shows us that one of the main ways that a cell lets something in and out of the body is by changing its *polarity,* or its electrical current. There is a specific voltage inside and outside the cell that can be changed by a number of factors and can be measured by various devices. For example, we have the ability to change our electrical potential when we relax or we get stressed. Humans work within a range of energy vibration, and these ranges are determined by specific centers in the body. They are like the control centers on the system of electrical energy flowing within the body. These are the same "highways" or "channels" targeted by acupuncture, an ancient healing practice of inserting needles to remove blocks or stagnation. The energy centers in the body have been categorized in diverse ways, such as nerve clusters, according to modern medicine and physics. New Age systems of thought and healing often use the phrase "energy centers" to refer to these same junctions. Some historians contend that Ayurveda is the oldest medical tradition from which all other medical systems were derived. Ayurveda refers to the energy vibration centers of the human being as *chakras,* or spinning wheels.

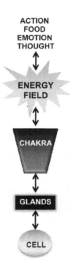

We all have chakras. We may not be aware of them. However, if we are conscious of them, they are excellent gauges of how we are responding to our environment on a subtle level. Within the chakras is the universal flux of consciousness, including archetypal information, so the complexity of the chakras and of what they provide to us if we tap into them is truly remarkable.

Very simply, the chakras are the basic foundation of our soul, connecting it to all layers of our being, including our physical body. They serve as points of integration for our physical, emotional, mental, and spiritual selves. Chakras have been recognized for thousands of years by ancient civilizations in Asia and South America. In particular, Indian yogic literature addresses these subtle energy centers. My experience with chakras is that they can be perceived as light and color and are often associated with images, either symbolic or literal in interpretation. Some individuals perceive chakras as wheels, spiraling in energy from the collective consciousness into the inner core of the physical body and vice versa. Traditional literature states that the chakra structure is a cone-shaped vortex vertically aligned at specific points from the base of the spine to the top of the head, transforming and transmitting the incoming finer energy into the more dense physical energy of the body.

In addition to the wheel image, chakras have also been associated with the symbol of a flower, with each chakra higher up the body (the head being the highest) having a relatively greater number of petals than the previous. The increasing complexity of the chakras moving from the lower to the higher parts of the body symbolizes the evolution from the material to the nonmaterial and from lower to higher consciousness.

According to Richard Gerber, M.D., in *Vibrational Medicine,* these important chakra centers have been discarded by Western scientists as "magical constructs of unsophisticated and primitive Eastern thinkers." The existence of chakras, or at least of the subtle energy field, has not been validated directly by scientific methods or devices. There are various machines on the market to measure one's energy field by placing your hand on a panel, reading the electric charge, and correlating the charge with energy channels (referred to in traditional Chinese medicine as "meridians") in the body. Although still slow in coming, the evidence for the existence of chakras has been initiated by various researchers such as Dr. Hiroshi Motoyama and Dr. Valerie Hunt, using technology designed to measure subtle energy. These are promising attempts that will propel us forward into doing more work in this area from a scientific perspective.

Quantum physics, seemingly more than any other scientific discipline, has provided us with support for the existence of the human energy field as a dynamic pattern of weblike interconnectedness. In the meantime, more practical means of accessing the chakras could come from indirect data, such as an individual's emotional and physical issues.

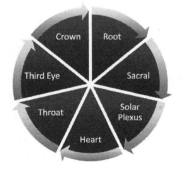

A majority of texts and philosophical systems agrees that there are seven major chakras and a multitude of minor chakras (some sources say up to 360). In this book, we work with the seven major chakras only. These chakras regulate key functions and issues and correspond to seven distinct anatomical areas (see Table 2.1). Since the chakras are central to the functioning of the body, symptoms or disease often begin in the chakras before moving into physical form. All thoughts, emotions, and actions are stored in our bodies. The chakras are a part of that process.

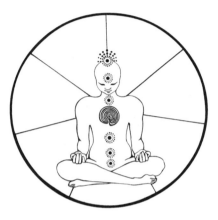

Table 2.1   Chakra Names, Locations, and Colors

Chakra Number	Chakra Name	Body Location	Corresponding Color	Element
1	Root	Base of spine, genital area	Red, brown, black	Earth
2	Sacral	Below the navel and above the pubic bone	Orange	Water
3	Solar Plexus	Upper middle abdomen	Yellow	Fire
4	Heart	Heart, below shoulders	Green, pink	Air
5	Throat	Neck, mouth, nose, ears	Turquoise	Ether
6	Third Eye	Between eyebrows	Indigo, purple	Light
7	Crown	Top of head	Lavender, white	Consciousness

When the chakras get overloaded with a negative message, the chakra may get blocked, and eventually the energy flow will be impeded in this area, causing symptoms or a disease in the organs that chakra is responsible for. You will learn more specifics as you read the chapters that correspond to the individual chakras. For example, if an individual has symptoms related to his or her stomach, then the solar plexus chakra should be addressed. A blockage in the heart chakra may suggest heart disease. Similarly, an individual who presents symptoms of adrenal stress would have issues to process in the root chakra.

COLOR AND VIBRATION

Have you ever thought to yourself that a certain person had a "bad vibe"? You were most likely tuning into their energy vibration. Every person carries an overall vibration reflecting the sum of the individual chakra vibrations. This vibration is the accumulation of the cell vibrations as the macrocosm (the individual) reflects the microcosm (the cells). The chakras are the "middle man" or collective center to which all the cells associated with that chakra report so that the chakra vibrates at that level. Each chakra will have a slightly different vibration, depending on its function and location.

Usually, a specific color is associated with the chakra, since color is, in fact, simply a physical manifestation of a vibration. The entire rainbow spectrum of colors is carried collectively within the seven chakras. Each chakra is associated with and responsible for a color resonating with its vibration; however, that does not mean that each chakra is limited to one color only. The color of a chakra will give information about the state of the chakra and its vibration. An easy way to remember the color associations is to think about the colors in a rainbow starting from the bottom upward (root chakra: red to crown chakra: lavender).

CHAKRAS AND THEIR ELEMENTS

The chakras are connected to color, archetypes, and also the elements of nature and the cosmos. Each chakra embodies some aspect of an element, with the lower body chakras taking on significantly "coarser" physical elements than the upper body chakras, which integrate elements that are not apparent to the naked eye. The root (first) chakra, with its association to being grounded and stable, appropriately carries the solid energy of the Earth and all her embodiments: soil, deep molten lava, rock. The sacral (second) chakra represents the water element, taking on its fluid, dynamic ability to create through life, being yielding and passive, yet strong and forceful at the same time. The solar plexus (third) chakra signifies the fire element, powerful and ready to ignite with confidence and the quality of "presence." These three chakras carry within their energies the symbolism and characteristics of physical elements (Earth, water, and fire). As you will read further, this association parallels their connection with these same elements found in the major components (macronutrients) comprising foods: the **root chakra** and its anchor to **earth** through **protein;** the **sacral chakra** capturing the movement inherent within **water** through its resonance with **fluids and fats;** and the **solar plexus** chakra honoring the **fire** quality of **carbohydrates,** a fuel source that is preferentially burned for energy in its variety of forms (everything from quick simple sugars to sustained complex starches).

As we travel up the chakra circuit into the upper body chakras, the elements become less tangible and more ethereal. The heart (fourth) chakra draws us to the elemental essence of air, which allows us to be part of the human experience. We can do for weeks without food, days without water, but only minutes without air. Ancient traditions revere the breath, or oxygen, and equate it with being our life force (*chi, prana*). Think of the word *in-spire,* which in Latin means "to breathe." We relate it to becoming exalted and infused with emotion and nourished. The throat (fifth) chakra's element is even finer than air—ether, the element of the heavens, or that space beyond the Earth. We communicate to the heavens and move beyond into space by air flowing through our throat chakra, creating sound, a vibration that travels through Earth gases, solids, and liquids into the substance that envelops the Earth. Up in the realm of the third eye (sixth) chakra resides the multidimensional element of light, or photonic, rainbowed particles and waves. This center provides our insight, or "lights the path" before us. Physiologically, it is very sensitive to the rhythms of light appearance and disappearance. It feeds off of the sunlight and the Divine light that shines from within everyone. Finally, the crown (seventh) links us to the element of oneness and wholeness of Divine energy and universal consciousness. It is the complete part of who we are and with this element in place, our bodies, minds, hearts, and souls are sustained.

CHAKRA HEALTH

A healthy chakra will be responsive to both internal cell messages and to external environment signals. It will open and close, like a flower responding to sunlight, bringing in and releasing energy, and creating an overall movement that translates into a vibration. Chakras take in energy or signals and direct them to the appropriate body systems. Health is determined by this flow of energy from the chakras through the energy circuits and into the metabolic network of the body. For example, if your boss tells you what a good job you are doing, your root chakra, responsible for survival and trust, may take in the message and create a supportive vibration. The root chakra is connected to the other chakras to give them this message, spreading the vibration throughout the body, allowing each chakra to filter what it needs to take in.

A chakra can also become blocked or obstructed, causing the internal or external messages to not get through or to become distorted. If we take the example of the boss's message, an unhealthy root chakra may distort the message and construe it as "The boss has been watching me" or further to "My job is in jeopardy," especially when the foundation of the root chakra has fear as one of its layers. Alternately, a child could receive a message from his parents at a very young age that children are to be seen and not heard. Such a message could create a block or a shutting down of the throat chakra, responsible for personal expression and truth speaking. Therefore, external input can make our chakras unhealthy, and it can also add to the dysfunction of the chakra. Sometimes, we have messages passed down to us from our DNA. These can be more challenging, since they are more hardwired than our immediate environmental input. However, with the proper healing tools and techniques, we can heal ourselves. Part of the journey to do so requires that we believe we can.

Malfunctioning chakras can become deficient or excessive in energy.

Malfunctioning chakras can become deficient or excessive in energy. When a chakra is clogged, it means that the upward energy flow to that center has become congested or stopped. Since the chakras act as spinning wheels, dispersing energy throughout the body, blocked chakras can restrict the entire energy flow to that area. Blockages often correspond to emotional, mental, and/or spiritual issues. For example, grief or anger could lodge in the heart chakra, giving rise to heart disease. Low esteem and anger could impact the solar plexus chakra, causing digestive complaints.

Chakras are energy deficient due to either a blockage or depletion of energy into that center—that is, the chakra is not being nourished by *chi* or *prana* to the extent that is required for adequate functioning. One simple, basic approach to restoring energy is to work on the center directly, using a variety of methods, including specific foods, dietary supplements, and lifestyle changes. The idea is to restore the vibration of the chakra with an external source that carries that same vibration or higher. Sometimes, stimulation of the chakra with physical touch (for example, acupressure, hands-on healing) is effective for releasing blocked energy. Chakras can also be restored by altering thought and emotional patterns.

Chakras can hold and process excessive energy, usually due to a blockage in the chakras above or below them or from external circumstances. Therefore, the chakras work in a domino-like fashion. They are interconnected to each other, and as a result a change in one chakra commonly influences the others in varying degrees. One way to balance energy into an overactive site is to work on spreading the energy to the chakras above or below it through foods, meditation, visualization, and so on. If there is overactivity in the sacral chakra, for example, it could be balanced if the chakra below (root chakra) and above it (solar plexus chakra) were worked on as well. Often, the higher chakra is stimulated in order to reduce the activity of the lower one, since energy tends to travel upward. In the case of the overactive sacral chakra, it may be best to work primarily on the solar plexus chakra.

All the chakras relate to each other in a weblike manner. However, they form particular groupings. The typical connection between the chakras is that the root chakra (first) is supported by the solar plexus (third) chakra. The solar plexus chakra, in turn, is supported by the throat (fifth) chakra, which is ultimately supported by the crown (seventh) chakra. In a similar fashion, the sacral (second) chakra has an intimate relationship with the heart (fourth) chakra, which then connects with the third eye (sixth) chakra. Therefore, an issue of an overactive heart chakra would best be addressed by working on the third eye chakra and supporting the sacral chakra. The odd-numbered and even-numbered chakras are special individual circuits: the odd-numbered chakras represent the masculine part of us, encompassing the dynamics of tribe, power, and expression; and the even-numbered chakras reflect the feminine aspects of our being, including emotions, sensuality, giving and receiving, and intuition.

The chakras work in a domino-like fashion. They are interconnected to each other, and as a result a change in one chakra commonly influences the others.

The energy field that surrounds our physical being is created by the collective vibration of all the chakras. It looks something similar to an egg shape around our entire body. This energy can be drained through leaks, tears, or energetic impurities in the fabric of our energy field. When this happens, there is a flaw in the functioning of the energetic field, leaving the individual with little energy to adequately support life. This effect cascades, negatively influencing the functioning of the chakras and ultimately the body. The flow of energy can also be irregular and disrupted from its normal paths locally or overall.

WORKING WITH THE CHAKRAS

The chakra system provides a convenient way for us to make our way to the internal, finer workings of our delicate, intricate beings. Through an understanding of the chakras, we can develop inner unity, balance, and peace, which will ultimately help us to grasp our surroundings and the larger universe. According to East Indian texts and newer Western methods, typical approaches to accessing these centers include crystals, meditations, visualizations, and yoga. In this book, we use a questionnaire (in chapter 3) to help you identify areas of your chakra system that may require healing. There is much information stored within these centers, so as one begins to work on the issues related to chakras through foods, it is likely that emotional issues will begin to surface to facilitate the healing of those centers.

THE FOOD-CHAKRA CONNECTION

So how do we make the leap from chakras, our vital energy centers, containing the essence of everything we are and will be, to something physical like food? How do we use foods to heal every aspect of ourselves? Embedded within the food are many kinds of information that feed us. When we eat, we take in and assimilate what the food has to offer. If you want to assess how a particular food will affect your energetic self, first identify its obvious characteristics: where it is grown, how it grows, its external and internal colors, whether it is solid or liquid or both. From there you can go deeper into pinpointing its nutrient composition: Is it primarily carbohydrate, fat, or protein? The culmination of all these aspects will ripple through our physical body to impact the vibration of our chakras and the flow of energy running through the chakras.

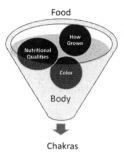

Food

Think about it in simplistic, familiar terms: We are energy. Food is energy. On a certain occasion, perhaps we literally feel "low on energy" because we have been working extra hours and taking on additional responsibilities. Certain foods may embody optimal physical qualities that give us the physical nourishment to feel revived. On another level, this food may capture within it the vibration that is needed to repair and correct spiritual patterns in our solar plexus chakra (responsible for our energy input and output), so that we will choose not to let ourselves get into situations where we know that our energy will be drained. One such example of a food that would perform both of these functions would be whole grains. On a physical level, whole grains contain a blend of mostly carbohydrate (mainly starches and fibers), some protein, and a small amount of fat. Complex carbohydrates like starches provide our bodies with a gradual release of energy in the form of sugar so that we could sustain our energy over time.

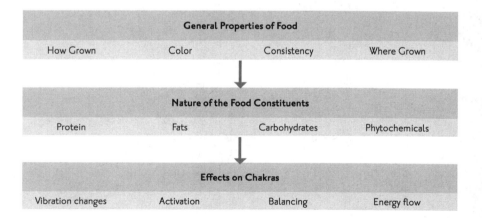

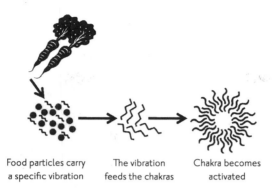

Food particles carry   The vibration   Chakra becomes
a specific vibration   feeds the chakras   activated

If we look at the physical qualities of the food, they reveal to us aspects of its spiritual messages. In the case of the whole grain, note that the essence of the plant, the germ, is tightly encased by the endosperm (or middle, starchy) layer and then protected further by the bran (outer) coating. In energetic terms, this plant speaks to us of protecting our essence from depletion.

Now if we ate processed grains repeatedly, we might experience the opposite of this phenomenon. First, processed grains will be lower in long chains of sugars and higher in simple sugars, ultimately leading to a rapid influx of sugar into the bloodstream. Therefore, we get a strong, initial spike of energy due to the fast release of sugar, but because of the corresponding quick release of insulin to shuttle the sugar into the cells, we end up with low blood sugar or hypoglycemia. Signs of low blood sugar include shakiness, headache, and fatigue. Our energy is depleted. Instead of enriching ourselves with energy from the food matrix, on an energy level we have made the process of eating a very costly one. Furthermore, the spiritual essence of a processed grain indicates a lack of integration and structure. Processed grains typically lack the germ and bran layer, leaving only the starchy endosperm. The spiritual message we send to our cells is one of a lack of wholeness and cohesion, causing us to disperse our energy.

Another example of how food can feed us spiritually is through color. In the instance with low energy, yellow foods can be stimulating and balancing to the solar plexus chakra, since they would transmit the vibration of yellow to the chakra. The solar plexus chakra is balanced when vibrating at the resonance of the color yellow. Thus, eating the spice curry would be very vibrationally congruent with this energy center and provide the solar plexus with the color frequency it needs. The curry compounds also stimulate physiological digestion through their warming nature. As a result, curry feeds the energy center through its color and its inherent physical properties.

As we go through each of the chakras in chapters 4 through 10, you will read about more of these physical-spiritual properties of food and how they may help you to work with specific challenges. When we learn to use foods and to eat in alignment with our soul, the healing begins. Increased consciousness occurs when all our many aspects are aligned and connected. Think of a boat with many oars going in all directions, but once they are aligned on one path, the boat flows forward at full speed. Such is the relationship with our spiritual selves. Our soul is the culmination and interconnection of many layers of varying vibration, with the densest one being the body, or physical layer.

In the next chapter we provide a questionnaire that asks about your physiological, emotional, and mental states. By completing the questionnaire you will be able to uncover which chakra(s) need support from food and eating. Afterward, you can read chapters 4 through 10 straight through or jump to the chapter that best addresses the chakra you would like to work on.

CHAPTER 3

DISCOVERING YOUR
CHAKRA ISSUES

*If you always do what you've always done,
you'll always get what you've always gotten.*
—ANTHONY ROBBINS

In this chapter, you will be able to identify the chakra issues that require healing by completing a questionnaire that integrates our physiological, emotional, and spiritual aspects. At the end of each section of the questionnaire, you will add up your score for that section. The highest scores indicate the direction of the chakra imbalances. It is common to find that there is more than one chakra that needs repair. In that case, it is recommended to address the lowest-number chakra first, since a block in a lower chakra will most likely turn into a blockage in the higher chakras. (Remember that, for the most part, energy in the body flows upward.) Your results will point you to the chapters that address each of the chakras individually.

I recommend completing this questionnaire in a quiet place, and as honestly as possible. You can also use the questionnaire to track your progress in the future, as you work through these issues using food as your healing tool.

CHAKRA QUESTIONNAIRE

The questionnaire is divided into seven sections, one for each chakra. For each of the fifteen questions within each section, read each statement and rate, from I to 5, how much it applies to you. Then, add up your scores from each section, giving you a total of seven scores at the end. The highest score will denote which chakra is most unbalanced in you. Let's say your sacral chakra has the greatest number of points. In this case, you could flip to the chapter on the sacral chakra (chapter 5) to read more about nourishing this chakra with foods.

Some of the questions relate to your physical body and may be more obvious than the questions on your emotions and thoughts. For the more subjective questions, try to answer how you have felt and acted for at least the past month.

Section I: Root Chakra
I = Does Not Apply   3 = Applies Sometimes   5 = Applies All the Time

1. Most times I do not feel safe or I feel that my boundaries are violated.
    1 2 3 4 5

2   I suffer from lack of energy and constant fatigue. 1 2 3 4 5

3. It is difficult to survive in this world. 1 2 3 4 5

4   Sometimes I feel like life isn't worth the effort. 1 2 3 4 5

5. I have a hard time sticking up for myself. 1 2 3 4 5

6. I lack initiative and may appear "lazy" to others. 1 2 3 4 5

7. For whatever reason(s), I am unable to be a part of a community and feel good about it. 1 2 3 4 5

8. My childhood left me feeling unloved. 1 2 3 4 5

9. Sometimes I resist and even despise family traditions and refuse to take part in them. 1 2 3 4 5

10. I am either physically or emotionally disconnected from my family of origin. 1 2 3 4 5

11. I frequently catch myself being spaced out or daydreaming, like I am not in my body. 1 2 3 4 5

12. Whenever a cold or flu is in the air, I am one of the first people to get it.
    1 2 3 4 5

13. (*For men*) Impotence is a concern for me. 1 2 3 4 5

14. I feel unprotected, like I have to "watch my back." 1 2 3 4 5

15. I struggle with my body image. 1 2 3 4 5

    Root Chakra Total: _____

Section 2: Sacral Chakra

I = Does Not Apply   3 = Applies Sometimes   5 = Applies All the Time

1. My body has difficulty regulating fluids (for example, I tend to urinate often; I am prone to swelling in my hands and ankles). 1 2 3 4 5
2. I've struggled to make money or to save it. 1 2 3 4 5
3. I have little interest in following through on ideas. 1 2 3 4 5
4. Eating fish is unappetizing for me. 1 2 3 4 5
5. I am an "emotional eater." 1 2 3 4 5
6. I have suffered from a severe emotional trauma at some point in my life that I have difficulty overcoming. 1 2 3 4 5
7. I have allowed myself to be (emotionally, physically) abused by others. 1 2 3 4 5
8. I often feel guilty, especially about my food choices. 1 2 3 4 5
9. There is (are) relationships that I've been in that I have not been able to recover from. 1 2 3 4 5
10. (*Women only*) I have health issues with my reproductive organs (for example, uterus, ovaries). 1 2 3 4 5
11. I prefer being alone rather than being with others, or I cannot tolerate being alone. 1 2 3 4 5
12. I see myself as either an overly creative or noncreative person. 1 2 3 4 5
13. I have challenges around expressing my sexuality, or I express my sexuality too freely. 1 2 3 4 5
14. Conveying my emotions to others is difficult. 1 2 3 4 5
15. Commitment to a project or a relationship can be a challenge for me. 1 2 3 4 5

   Sacral Chakra Total: _____

Section 3: Solar Plexus Chakra

I = Does Not Apply   3 = Applies Sometimes   5 = Applies All the Time

1. Achievement of a goal is very important to me. 1 2 3 4 5
2. I exhaust myself by thinking too much. 1 2 3 4 5
3. I would call myself overstressed. 1 2 3 4 5
4. Saying "No" to people is difficult for me. 1 2 3 4 5

5. I don't do well when presented with many choices. 1 2 3 4 5
6. I crave high-energy foods to keep me going. 1 2 3 4 5
7. I would say that I am addicted to sugar. 1 2 3 4 5
8. I suffer from digestive complaints, mainly indigestion and bloating.
   1 2 3 4 5
9. I need external substances (food, drugs, alcohol) to help me relax.
   1 2 3 4 5
10. My weight fluctuates often. 1 2 3 4 5
11. I tend to be a perfectionist. 1 2 3 4 5
12. After I have been around other people, I feel drained of energy.
    1 2 3 4 5
13. I lack self-confidence, or I have an inflated sense of confidence.
    1 2 3 4 5
14. I find myself worrying about what others will think of me. 1 2 3 4 5
15. Most people would call me analytical, and maybe even critical.
    1 2 3 4 5

Solar Plexus Chakra Total : _____

Section 4: Heart Chakra

1 = Does Not Apply   3 = Applies Sometimes   5 = Applies All the Time

1. My moods change often and I tend to be melodramatic. 1 2 3 4 5
2. I rarely have a chance to do what is best for me, or I tend to be overly
   selfish. 1 2 3 4 5
3. I neglect to eat green vegetables. 1 2 3 4 5
4. My hands get cold easily. 1 2 3 4 5
5. I am anxious. 1 2 3 4 5
6. Only select people are allowed to be close to me, physically or
   emotionally. 1 2 3 4 5
7. I have not felt true joy or happiness in recent years. 1 2 3 4 5
8. I feel shut down from my deepest feelings. 1 2 3 4 5
9. For the most part, my decisions are purely intellectual. 1 2 3 4 5
10. I have some form of heart disease (for example, atherosclerosis, arterio-
    sclerosis, heart failure, heart attack, high cholesterol). 1 2 3 4 5
11. If I let myself cry, I feel that I may not be able to stop. 1 2 3 4 5
12. I lack passion for anything in life. 1 2 3 4 5

13. I find it difficult to touch or to be touched. 1 2 3 4 5
14. A traumatic event in my life has caused me to be unable to connect with my emotions. 1 2 3 4 5
15. I have issues receiving or giving love. 1 2 3 4 5

Heart Chakra Total: _____

Section 5: Throat Chakra

1 = Does Not Apply   3 = Applies Sometimes   5 = Applies All the Time

1. My verbal expression has been limited or excessive. 1 2 3 4 5
2. It is not my nature to speak up when I have been wrongfully accused.
   1 2 3 4 5
3. I have chewing or swallowing difficulties. 1 2 3 4 5
4. Speaking my personal truth has not come easy. 1 2 3 4 5
5. My voice becomes raspy and my throat dry when I try to speak something I feel strongly about. 1 2 3 4 5
6. My metabolism is too slow or too fast. 1 2 3 4 5
7. Either I talk too much or I am afraid to speak for fear of being punished.
   1 2 3 4 5
8. I have thyroid problems. 1 2 3 4 5
9. I've dealt with eating disorders (for example, anorexia, bulimia).
   1 2 3 4 5
10. It is easier for me to write my feelings than to speak them. 1 2 3 4 5
11. My hearing and sense of smell are either deadened or heightened.
   1 2 3 4 5
12. Surrendering to a Higher Power is a difficult concept for me.
   1 2 3 4 5
13. Praying is not something I feel comfortable doing. 1 2 3 4 5
14. I tend to agree with others rather than create any discord. 1 2 3 4 5
15. My opinion is less or more important than the harmony of a group.
   1 2 3 4 5

Throat Chakra Total: _____

Section 6: Third Eye Chakra

I = Does Not Apply   3 = Applies Sometimes   5 = Applies All the Time

1. My life purpose is unclear. I   2   3   4   5
2. I am prone to depression. I   2   3   4   5
3. My dreams can either be nightmarish and vivid or I can rarely remember them. I   2   3   4   5
4. My mind often goes blank or is cluttered with random thoughts.
    I   2   3   4   5
5. I feel out of touch with my intuition. I   2   3   4   5
6. My needs for sleep seem to be very different from what most people need. I   2   3   4   5
7. I cannot go without caffeine. I   2   3   4   5
8. I tend to live inside my own mind and find myself daydreaming often.
    I   2   3   4   5
9. My eyesight is diminished. I   2   3   4   5
10. Drugs are a part of my life or were a part of my recent past. I   2   3   4   5
11. This life feels unreal for me, almost illusory, and I have difficulty staying present. I   2   3   4   5
12. My tendency is to get away from it all in whatever ways I can.
    I   2   3   4   5
13. I get strong chocolate cravings. I   2   3   4   5
14. I have abused or abuse alcohol, particularly hard liquor and wine.
    I   2   3   4   5
15. I am overly concerned with other realities. I   2   3   4   5

Third Eye Chakra Total: _____

Section 7: Crown Chakra

I = Does Not Apply   3 = Applies Sometimes   5 = Applies All the Time

1. I lack faith in a Higher Power, or I am overzealous in conveying my religious beliefs. I   2   3   4   5
2. I tend to be resentful of others who are overreligious or very forthright in their beliefs about God. I   2   3   4   5
3. I lack a specific belief system about my connection with all of life.
    I   2   3   4   5
4. I feel let down by a Higher Power. I   2   3   4   5
5. I have spiritual beliefs that I neglect to live by. I   2   3   4   5

6. I avoid an intimate connection with God for fear that it would change my life. 1 2 3 4 5

7. I struggle to maintain faith in living. 1 2 3 4 5

8. My experience with life has left me feeling that something is missing. 1 2 3 4 5

9. Life only goes so deep. 1 2 3 4 5

10. My body and spirit feel disconnected. 1 2 3 4 5

11. I doubt that I would be helped by a Higher Power in the event that I would need assistance. 1 2 3 4 5

12. I do not pray. 1 2 3 4 5

13. My spiritual views are nonexistent. 1 2 3 4 5

14. I search for a greater meaning to my life and do not seem to find anything satisfying. 1 2 3 4 5

15. I often feel lost in my life. 1 2 3 4 5

Crown Chakra Total: _____

Chakra Score Summary: _____

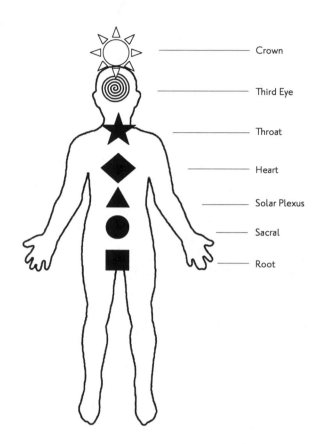

Crown

Third Eye

Throat

Heart

Solar Plexus

Sacral

Root

The chakra with the highest score indicates the greatest degree of imbalance. From here, you can either read the remainder of the book straight through, or you can skip to the chapter that addresses the chakra you most need to focus on as indicated by your score.

CHAPTER 4

FOODS FOR GROUNDING
AND PROTECTION

Feeding the Root Chakra

I think that what we're seeking is an experience of being alive,
so that our life experiences on the purely physical plane will
have resonances within our own innermost being and reality,
so that we actually feel the rapture of being alive.
—JOSEPH CAMPBELL

Earth • Roots • Grounding • Survival • Body •
Food • Matter • Beginning • Red • Square •
Tribe • Tradition • Abundance

LARRY: LOW ON GROUNDED ENERGY

Larry has mixed feelings about people. In the company of others, his identity wanes and he easily assumes the behavior and emotions of others. When he sees someone crying, his eyes well up with tears. If someone is angry, he feels rage swelling from within. As a result, Larry finds himself confused around other people. He is not sure what *he* actually feels. Being a taxi driver, around a wide variety of people, he comes home at the end of the day and feels "spaced out." Many times, his body collapses in fatigue. He responds best when he is able to exercise, such as lifting weights or running. Most of his free time is spent in seclusion so that his life feels less complicated.

Larry has spent much of his life in debt and has difficulty managing money. He hops from job to job, unable to make a significant commitment. He has resigned himself to jobs where he doesn't have to interface with the boss to any great level, as he finds himself resentful toward authority influences. Larry is constantly haunted by the thought of going broke and ending up on the street. Many of his family members are successful, and he feels that he could never rise to meet their level of accomplishment. Finally, Larry has issues committing to an intimate relationship, because at the core level he does not believe he is worthy of being loved.

Larry is the extreme example of someone who is ungrounded, or unable to cultivate a healthy experience on the physical level in the human flesh. His boundaries are weak, as he willingly takes on the feelings of those around him, rather than recognizing and centering in his own emotions and authentically experiencing the interaction with someone else. In a manner of speaking, he relies on others to assign him his identity without taking responsibility for his own feelings and thoughts. People such as Larry may have difficulty surviving in the daily world and believing in their right to exist. They are insecure, erratic, impatient, bored, and flighty. Common practices and activities such as holding a full-time job or balancing finances may present to them as uphill battles of strife and pain. Healing for Larry is about mining his internal worth and value so that he can express his emotions authentically as his own and earn money without fear.

THE ROOT CHAKRA: GROUNDING

UNHEALTHY ROOT CHAKRA INDICATIONS

Perhaps you feel as though you can identify with elements of Larry's situation. If you answer positively to the questions following, chances are you have issues with grounding and would benefit from some work on your root chakra.

- Do you feel like its "you" against "everyone else"?
- Do you find yourself trying to overcompensate by overachieving, overworking, and even overeating?

- Do you resist and even despise family traditions and refuse to take part in them?
- Are you at "war" with your family of origin?
- Are you suffering from inflammatory or autoimmune conditions?
- Do you sometimes feel like life isn't worth the effort?
- Do you feel that you are unloved and neglected by your family and friends, almost like you are invisible?
- Do you take special care to safeguard your possessions and yet you still feel unsafe, to the point where you feel like your life is in jeopardy?
- Do you often feel fatigued, like you can't go further?
- Do you frequently feel like you are separate from others around you, like you cannot seem to connect?

> **The ability to be grounded in the workings of the world on a physical level is a slow vibration, resonating stability, certainty, and physical strength.**

- Do you often feel spaced out, like you are "not in your body"?
- Do you frequently find yourself daydreaming, out of the moment?
- Do you feel that parts of your body are "breaking down," causing you to be unable to function optimally to earn your place in society?
- Do you constantly feel like you have to fight to defend yourself?
- Do you find that you second-guess yourself and your decisions, almost like you are battling from within?

HEALTHY ROOT CHAKRA BEHAVIOR

When our physical energy is functioning optimally, we will feel and know that we can survive adequately in this world. Even though there is truly no security because life is full of change and unpredictability, a healthy grounded person will feel on a core, deep level that he or she will always be provided for, whether through themselves, family, or society. These people are independent and determined, yet not afraid to confide in and depend on others if needed. Healthy grounded behavior means holding energy for an acceptance of family or tribe, whether actual (that is, blood relatives) or developed (that is, adopted family, marriage), and trust originates from the feeling of commitment to the tribe. Individuals who are grounded often have healthy boundaries, a strong feeling of their life purpose, and believe at their core that they have a right to exist or to be acknowledged as worthy. Other key words resonating with the healthy form of this physical energy include *commitment, purpose, patience, consistency,* and *security.*

THE SLOW VIBRATION OF PHYSICAL ENERGY

Why does it sometimes take so long to make a shift in our body, behaviors, actions, and thoughts? You can thank your root chakra for the slow steadiness of your change! Reflecting back to our discussion of vibrating matter or energy in earlier chapters, the ability to be grounded in the workings of the world on a physical level is a slow vibration, resonating stability, certainty, and physical strength. It is the foundation of our identity. To be grounded translates loosely into a feeling of being "with it" or "in tune" as it relates to a physical reality of performing tasks and engaging in activities. It encompasses a harmonious network of thinking, feeling, and sensing, revolving around being present in the physical world. When we acknowledge our physical form, our awareness of the surrounding environment is enhanced, making for fewer accidents and inefficiencies and, as a result, our life feels full and under control.

When we acknowledge our physical form, our awareness of the surrounding environment is enhanced, making for fewer accidents and inefficiencies and, as a result, our life feels full and under control.

This energy provides much of the framework on which the rest of our energy system is built. It could be compared to laying the physical foundation for the "house" of our energy and who we are. Without a firm foundation and established layers of trust, security, and safety, we can easily crumble when our other faster-moving vibrations are affected. As you will read later, the slow, grounded vibration is the "mother" of other vibrations carried within us to sustain our personal power (solar plexus chakra) and to express ourselves with the assistance of personal and Divine will (throat chakra).

WE ARE A LIVING ROOT OF ANCESTRY

Another way to view being grounded is to think of having a root or an anchor attached to the bottom of your feet. The human body is symbolically designed as a starlike structure. The two lower spokes, the legs, ending in the feet, make physical contact with the Earth. The two upper spokes, the arms, reach in the opposite direction of the heavens. Putting them together, we contain the balance of Earth and heaven within our structure.

It is important for us to *feel* and *connect* with our pelvic shell, harboring our sacrum and our reproductive organs (men), as well as with the long stretch of legs and feet. For most people, the feet are the only part of us that physically contacts the Earth for a majority of the day—a fraction of the expanse of our body! Through our feet, we can transmit the Earth's slow, steady vibration upward into our structure, allowing it to nourish us and to enable us to be comfortable with being Earthbound.

On a larger, more cosmic scale, ancestral energies live within the dense root chakra vibration. Cultures like those that are Shamanic in origin hold tight to their traditions and lineage. As a result, they are closely tied to the root chakra energy. If we choose to look very deeply at our origins, we will find that every single past event creates our being. We are the cumulative sum of our ancestral and individual energies, spiraling together, forming the matrix of our outer body shell. Our bodies are testament to this memory. We reflect who we have been and who we have chosen to be by our selection into our tribe. Every moment of our personal history has been perfectly crafted. The memory of the past is found within every cell in the human body, encased within the strands of DNA. So, when we hear the phrase, "It's in your genes," we are really talking about our connection to ancient cellular memory. This vibration carries with it the foundations of physical life and needs of survival, including core issues relating to family, food, shelter, sexuality, safety, and trust. There is no doubt that we are wired for survival.

THE NATURE OF THE GROUNDED VIBRATION

The slow vibration of grounded earthliness that is a part of our being often resonates with the color red, like the rich, scarlet color of blood. Blood connects us with our lineage, our ancestors. However, other colors, such as black, charcoal gray, and dark brown, colors of the moist, loamy soil and clay of the Earth layers, are also associated with this vibration. The vibrations of our grounded self are slower than other aspects of our being, and as a result of this dense vibration, it typically takes relatively more time and work than the other vibrations we carry to heal or to change. The good side of this vibratory rate is that once change has been implemented, it can more readily stay strong and full and be difficult to imbalance.

Core Issues Associated with the Root Chakra

• Ability to defend oneself
• Ability to provide for life's necessities—to survive in the world
• Communal safety and security
• Familial and social law and order
• Feeling "at home" with self, family, and community
• Physical family

Many people place little emphasis and value on connecting with their earthly bodies and even disengage from it, causing them to appear flighty. However, it is worth remembering that grounding to the Earth through our being is essential for carrying out our life mission. We are spirit beings in a human body for a reason. Our dreams manifest with healthy grounded vibrations. Additionally, being grounded and feeling secure in our physical existence allows us to access a wealth of solutions for earthly matters by being more interactive with planetary life. We find valuable solutions by being in the present moment and grounded in our Earth experience.

PHYSIOLOGY AND THE ROOT CHAKRA

In addition to supporting our energetic structure, this slow, assured vibration provides the instinctual, primal template for who we are as physical human beings. It is responsible for the energy of body systems that provide us with physical structure, allowing us to make tangible, meaningful contact with the Earth. These anatomical parts include the joints, bones, muscle, legs, and feet. The root chakra also provides us with an internal and external defense system, including the immune system (internal "defense" strategy) and skin (external physical barrier between us and others), as a physical barrier to separate us as individuals from the environmental influences, or self from non-self. This defense system provides us with healthy boundaries.

Anatomy Associated with the Grounded Vibration

- Adrenal glands
- Blood cells (red and white)
- Bones
- DNA
- Feet
- Immune system
- Joints

- Legs
- Muscle
- Prostate gland
- Rectum
- Reproductive organs (male)
- Skin
- Tailbone (coccyx)

Adding to boundaries and defending the self are the adrenal glands. They are like the internal armor that provides us with the ability to "flee" or "fight" if we are in a situation that our life depends on. The adrenals give us that instinctual, primal urge to live no matter the cost and to make that decision instantaneously, as it is hardwired within us on the DNA level to survive. On a microcosm level, the grounded earthly vibration is embedded into the red and white blood cells, products of the bone marrow, and its essence is carried within every cell in the form of the double-stranded DNA that contains our genetic code.

Our DNA and immune system allow us to know who we are and are not. When we give up our need to connect to the Earth, we leave ourselves open to other influences. We become whatever flows into our physical, emotional, and mental space. The result is that we can feel disjointed, fragmented, and spread thin, similar to Larry. We exhaust our physical body resources because they are used up in guarding against invading influences that are not "self."

This grounded vibration solidifies in the genital area, where the legs meet. Therefore, it would govern the energy distributed to those parts of the anatomy residing in that terrain, including the prostate gland, male reproductive organs, and rectum. The vibrations of this center are particularly important for men, and are in part why some men connect their livelihood with their identity as potent beings, both financially and sexually. Some might say that a man's societal obligations and inherent masculinity reside in this vibration.

THE RELATIONSHIP OF GROUNDING
AND PROTECTION TO FOODS AND EATING

Since the root chakra focuses primarily on the layer of us that needs basic elements for survival, it is no wonder that this center is tied closely to our relationship with the key essentials that we confront on a daily basis for physiological function several times a day—*food and eating*. Therefore, it is not surprising that many of our food issues are harbored within the realm of this chakra.

ROOT CHAKRA FOOD AND EATING HEALING PLAN

Feel Secure about Accessing Food

Maslow's hierarchical triangle speaks of our basic needs serving the foundation of our being. Without air, food, and water, we are without life. Money provides the abundance to be able to access food. The way we "earn a living" and our feelings about money are directly related to our root chakra: if this area is blocked, stagnant, or closed down, we may operate from a place of lack, or an absence of abundance. With a cloudy root chakra filter, we may stamp people and situations in our lives with labels of "rich," "snobby," or "poor," creating an artificial boundary of limiting beliefs to rein us in from accessing the richness of abundance! When we believe along these lines, fear may surface in the purchase of food or meals. Someone who is stingy with money spent on meals may have a root chakra that requires healing.

On the other hand, if an individual is obsessive to the point of maximizing buffets and "getting their money's worth" from open selection of foods, this tendency could also point to root chakra imbalance. For example, in social settings, Jim will deliberately eat the remains left on everyone's plate at the end of a shared meal to ensure that all the food is gone and not wasted. The message of "eating everything on our plate" has resonated strongly within this culture, perhaps to the detriment of our root chakra. Similarly, within our culture, excessive large portions are encouraged. Look at the low prices to "supersize" in fast food places or the lower cost of buying in bulk quantities versus buying a few items. How do we interact with that message?

Coming from a large family where food was scarce, Jillian admits that she does not feel safe unless her pantry is completely stocked. Do we let the amount of food we eat or store determine our safety rather than cultivating that from within? Creating a healthy root chakra involves releasing ingrained fear messages about providing for food and knowing that you will always be able to access food when needed.

Eat When Hungry

In my opinion, one of the biggest problems with our modern society and our approach to eating is that we no longer rely on our body's inherent wisdom. Instead, we look to books on "how to eat" to tell us what we need. We ask the waitstaff at a restaurant what the best thing on the menu is. Sometimes we even give up our right to choose our foods by having others cook or order for us on a routine basis. Neglecting our body needs by refusing or denying ourselves foods indicates that the root chakra is at work. Self-inflicted starvation and anorexia, for example, are classic examples of instances where the root chakra has been shut down to incoming life-promoting energy. As a result, the body form becomes almost nonexistent and withers to a willowy, thin shell. Food becomes an enemy rather than a nourishing, supportive substance. Individuals who refuse to eat have difficulty accepting that they have the "right to exist"—a major cornerstone of the root chakra.

Our root chakra contains the vibration of healthy physical hunger and being able to tap into that sensation when we feel called. When we ignore our body's hunger signals, our body gets the signal that it is not valued. A lack of trust develops. By dialoguing with our body about the foods it needs, we will be fulfilling our physical needs and satisfying our root chakra. The dialogue may be as simple as walking into your kitchen, feeling your toes on the floor to ground, and asking the "safe place" within you what you'd like to have. The idea of creating a safe place to go to within our body links us to our root chakra. I notice that it helps people to want to stay in their bodies. See what kinds of activities are happening in your safe place. During guided imageries, people report other sides of themselves like their inner child and a freer self that they do not feel safe to bring out in various contexts. When we practice this technique, the body and mind will develop a better trusting relationship, and eventually we will react appropriately to signals that our body is hungry rather than suppressing or ignoring them.

Another point is that so many people are so out of touch with their bodies that they are unable to distinguish between emotional and physical hunger. Physical hunger, originating from the gut, in contrast to emotional hunger, which springs from the mind, is a very distinct somatic signal that builds gradually and is open to a variety of food choices. Frequently, our body signals are not heard clearly enough because we do not pay attention.

Let Go of Protecting Oneself with Food

In our current society, more than 60 percent of the population has been categorized as overweight or obese. No apparent solution exists for this growing crisis. Of course, there are many contributors to excess body weight, including lifestyle behaviors such as eating poorly and remaining sedentary. However, if we look deeper to unearth the real causes at play, we may find that excess weight for some individuals may be linked to their inability to feel safe. The added weight provides padding and protection from attention. Julie admits that she started to gain weight as a teenager after people commented on the changes in her body and how attractive she was becoming. Her feelings of being scared and intimidated by the changes in her body manifested into overeating. During our nutrition consult, Julie reflects back to these comments, said to her some forty years ago, and is surprised at the power they continue to have over her. There is no question that they can grab hold of us.

Other clients have revealed to me that they have been physically or sexually abused in their lives, and as a result it feels safer to cover their body with excess so no one can see how attractive their body form is. So, excessive eating, much in the same way as abstinence from food, involves the energy of the root chakra. Too much eating can unground us to a similar extent as not eating at all. We numb ourselves when we take in too much food, causing ourselves to let go of feeling. When we do not eat at all, we do not have the strength to feel, to process thoughts and emotions, and to be active. In both cases, we eject ourselves from our bodies through the button of food.

Instead of hiding ourselves in the shadow of too much food, we can use food to bring out the best of us—the vital, pure essence of who we are, basking in love. When we eat according to our body's needs, our mind remains sharp and our heart strong. We can focus on the moment and give attention to any thoughts, words, or actions that float in our sky of consciousness. The right amount of food for us in the moment hits the sweet spot of our consciousness. We feel alive and connected!

Engage in Healthy Social Eating

Social eating is a charged event. Most often, especially around the holidays, people tell me that they are conflicted by social eating events. Sometimes, they teeter on the stressful decision of whether to attend a gathering because of the foods that may be served. They find it fearful to "challenge the tribe" aspects of eating by saying no to eating certain foods. Lydia relays that at a party, a brownie was thrust into her mouth by a family member before she could say no. Later that day, she ended up with a throbbing migraine, as chocolate was one of her trigger foods. She was bedridden for hours. Even though she knew that this outcome would occur, she was unable to find internal strength within her root chakra to trust her own instinct and body. Of course, I advocate various strategies for dealing with challenging social aspects, such as eating beforehand, calling ahead of time to find out what will be served, and finally, participating in the tribal preparation of a meal by bringing a dish! Potlucks are healthy root chakra events for all involved!

FOODS FOR GROUNDING AND PROTECTION

Foods for grounding and protection are rooted in physical form. Their vibration quality is represented by a square shape, a solid, foundational structure, similar to that of a house. These foods assist us in reestablishing and strengthening our connection to the earthly vibration within us, bringing us back to our root. These foods make us feel heavy and slower moving, quite possibly a welcome feeling when we live life by the seat of our pants! These grounding foods give us the "earthly substance" we need to keep our feet on the Earth and to make our dreams real and practical. They are ideal for enabling us to be centered and protected when we walk the line between distraction and vulnerability.

Choose lean, low-fat options for meat and animal products in order to maximize the amount of protein for grounding. Highly concentrated protein foods such as eggs, meat, or milk are solidifying and have a stabilizing effect on one's grounding energy.

Protein

In the nutrition universe, protein is the nutrient that gives us our structure and the raw materials to ground and anchor the body to the Earth. The building blocks of proteins ("amino acids") are contained throughout the physical structure of our being, such as in muscle, bone, and the immune system. If we zoom in closer to the cell level, we will see that proteins are responsible for many of the minute happenings within the cell, such as catalyzing reactions and maintaining cell shape and growth. They serve as the chief implementers of whatever information is encoded in the gene headquarters.

Of the twenty or so amino acids that exist and are arranged in proteins in various combinations, about eight of these are considered essential for our existence, implying that our physical bodies cannot manufacture these on their own. Therefore, they must be eaten. A full complement of the essential amino acids is found in animal foods. Some foundational grounding high-protein foods include eggs and milk. Think of the nature of an egg from a hen. If the egg were fertilized, it would have all the necessary nutritional constituents for nourishing the growth of the chick embryo, similar to the function of the root chakra. The very appearance of the egg, with the yellow yolk surrounded by the shiny, pearled-white orb suggests that it imparts a protective nature from an archetypal, symbolic standpoint. Hard-boiled eggs make very good additions in a routine as a mid-morning or mid-afternoon snack, as they allow us to ground in the space between meals.

Animal-based foods are usually higher in quality, complete protein than most other vegetable-based foods. It is important to choose lean, low-fat options for meat and animal products in order to maximize the amount of protein for grounding. Highly concentrated protein foods such as eggs, meat, or milk are solidifying and have a stabilizing effect on one's grounding energy. In my experience, ungrounded individuals who fail to align their lives with their deep purpose do well on relatively higher protein (either animal or vegetable protein) diets until they are strengthened and centered. On the other hand, someone who is too stubborn and stuck in their ways requires *less* animal protein to help them release their strong grip on the Earth and to balance grounding, physical energy. Additionally, high amounts of grounding food can have a destabilizing, ungrounding effect. Eating too much turkey and drinking excessive warm milk, both very high-protein, root chakra-heavy foods, can lead to a sleepy sensation, as if one were removed from their reality into a dreamy, nonbody state. Therefore, keying into the level of grounding you require is essential for optimizing your dietary needs.

Once an ungrounded person has started working on her ability to be in physical harmony with the Earth by tuning into her physical body vibration, she will instinctually start craving high-protein animal foods. We cannot help but be drawn to these foods. I have had two clients whom I saw separately and who did not know each other, but they both ate buffalo on a regular basis and felt that they *needed* the buffalo meat. They were not willing to give it up. These individuals, both slight in stature, felt the need for the grounded nature of buffalo and the physical greatness and protective quality it carries. Conversely, someone who is overly grounded can crave a more vegetarian regimen. This association does not imply, however, that vegetarians are overly grounded. If someone with stuck root chakra energy continues to eat an excessively high-protein diet, increased production of uric acid can result, leading to its deposition in the extremities like the feet, otherwise known as gout. In this case, too much grounding leads to accumulation in the feet and pain, letting us know that we essentially have "too much connection" with the earthly vibration. This is one of many demonstrations of how our soul issues become our biology and vice versa. This indication demonstrates that our spiritual centers are in constant communication with us, if we are open to listening to their messages.

Despite the fact that it is easier to get high-quality proteins from animal-based foods, they can also be obtained from vegetable protein sources such as legumes, nuts, and seeds (see Table 4.1). Usually, a combination of vegetable foods, such as the famous rice-and-beans duo, is needed to get the same amino acid spectrum. Specifically, this combination is superb for anchoring both the root and solar plexus chakras. However, complementing vegetable protein is not always needed. Some, like soy, are grounded enough to stand alone. Under recent accepted guidelines to determine protein digestibility, soy protein has been assessed to be as complete a protein as milk protein.

Scientific literature and overall public health recommendations have detailed the numerous benefits of vegetable protein over animal protein for indications such as heart disease and cancer, to name a few. Personally, I like vegetable protein as a constant grounding baseline for most individuals. Some folks may prefer and feel drawn to animal protein for various reasons, including imparting to them the grounded vibration. It is best to be in tune with your body to read these needs specifically. Many people seem to feel strongly about their choice source of protein, indicating the strong resonance of their root chakras.

Protein-containing foods are a staple of every meal in many countries. In fact, some cultures believe that a diet needs to contain meat in order for it to be "complete," an opinion that may be congruent with the need to ensure proper grounding for successful survival as a tribe. On a side note, the resurgence of the popularity of high-protein diets within the past five to seven years (it cycles through our eating culture) has been successful for so many people due to issues related to being ungrounded and unprotected, such as a loss of trust and safety. It follows good logic that high-protein diets would become a trend, especially after experiencing a jolt in our ability to root ourselves after the nationwide devastation of September 11, 2001. As a result of this calamity, Americans experienced increased fear and the threat of terrorism—a violation and breakdown of the safety and trust that reside in the slow-moving vibration of the body. High-protein diets come to the rescue to stabilize our need to feel safe and grounded in our bodies.

Table 4.1   Protein Levels of Selected Animal and Vegetable Foods

Food	Serving	Weight in Grams	Protein in Grams	Percentage Daily Value*
Almonds	I ounce	28.35	6.02	I2
Cheddar cheese	I ounce	28	7.I	I4
Chicken, roasted	6 ounces	I70	42.5	85
Egg	I large	50	6.3	I3
Hamburger, extra lean	6 ounces	I70	48.6	97
Lentils, cooked	$1/2$ cup	99	9	I8
Pumpkin seeds	I ounce	28.35	6.96	I3.9
Sunflower seeds	$1/4$ cup	35	7.27	I4.5
Tofu	$1/2$ cup	I26	I0.I	20
Tuna, water packed	6 ounces	I70	40.I	80
Yogurt, low-fat	8 ounces	227	II.9	24
Walnuts	I ounce	28.35	4.32	8.6

*Based on 2000 kcal

Source: Based on the USDA Nutrient Database values obtained at *http://www.nal.usda.gov/fnic/foodcomp/search/*

High-Protein Animal Foods to Ground and Protect

- Butter
- Buttermilk
- Cheese (hard, soft, cottage)
- Cream
- Eggs
- Ghee (clarified butter)
- Kefir
- Lean meats (beef, buffalo, chicken, lamb, ostrich, pork, turkey, veal, venison)
- Milk (cow, goat, sheep in origin)
- Yogurt

Eating primarily protein without a balance of the other macronutrients can literally make us too rigid, eventually leading to the breakdown of our root chakra structures. An excess of protein can lead to an imbalance of pH in the body systems, resulting in greater acidity. It is important to balance pH in the body, because numerous reactions in cells take place at specific pH ranges. For example, the enzymes to break down protein in the stomach function best at a low (acidic) pH, while the enzymes to break down starches in the small intestine work at a slightly alkaline pH. Greater acid milieu can throw the body out of balance and change the function of many organs. When there is high acid due to the intake of protein-rich foods (composed of amino *acids*), the body reads that as a signal to borrow from its precious alkaline reserves to normalize the levels. Where does the body have a high alkaline stock? The bones are high in alkalizing minerals such as calcium, magnesium, and phosphorus. So, in instances of increased body acidity, alkalizing minerals can be resourced from tissues like the bone, namely calcium, in order to bring the body back to a normal pH range. As a result, however, the bones become brittle and susceptible to breaking. In energy terms, we become less stable by throwing off the structural components of the body and the root chakra framework. Therefore, measuring urine pH periodically is a good way to test to see how acidic you are so that you can adjust your eating accordingly (ideal pH is close to 7). It is also an indirect way to see whether your grounding state is skewed.

Animal-Based Foods

Foods from animal origin are some of the *most* effective food tools when grounding and protection are needed, especially animals that are land based, with four feet consistently in contact with the Earth. Four-footed animals reflect the square symbolism behind grounded foods and provide us two-legged creatures with extra support. Perhaps it is not surprising that animals contribute their solid, grounded energy when in their presence or when we take in their flesh as food since they are so proficient at staying in the moment, living according to their instinctual selves in harmony with the Earth. We are able to merge with this vibration in order to help protect our identity and to feel and find comfort with ourselves in the web of life on Earth. Physiologically, our bodies take longer to digest flesh foods because they are dense, suggesting that they stay in our bowels for an extended time, creating a grounded, full feeling deep in the gut. However, if we are too grounded in this reality, these types of animal foods can leave us feeling uncomfortably full, stuck, and lethargic, thus having the reverse effect.

It is worthwhile to mention that the different four-legged animals carry their own distinct energy vibration layered on top of the grounded energy they exude. We take on the energy of that particular animal when we are in its presence or eat its flesh. For example, a cow provides grounded energy that is serene and complacent, whereas the grounded energy of a sheep encourages community and sharing (see Table 4.2). Therefore, I recommend cow-derived food products to someone who is high-strung and distracted and sheep-based foods to individuals who feel isolated and vulnerable.

Like meat, the vibration of the animal is woven into the products made from these animals, such as milk, yogurt, or cheese, although probably not to the same intensity as eating the meat of the animal since there is more processing and manipulation by humans or machines. Milk has a complete nutritional profile, with the correct ratios of protein, carbohydrate, and fat for the growing calf. In addition to the nutritional building blocks for growth it contains, it also carries the vibration for the support of a foundation for life. Milk is not a common food that I recommend to clients, as many people are either sensitive or allergic to it, or are lactose intolerant. However, in small amounts, at times

Table 4.2   Characteristics of Four-Legged Land-Based Animal Foods

Animal	Specific Characteristics
Buffalo	Wisdom, ancestral knowledge, protection
Cow	Serenity, peace, justice
Goat	Endurance, courage, accomplishment
Lamb	Gentleness, kindness
Ostrich	Pride, independence, morality
Pig	Loyalty, honesty, forgiveness
Sheep	Sense of community, sharing
Turkey	Gratitude, objectivity, generosity
Venison (includes deer, moose, elk, caribou, antelope)	Compassion, guidance, warmheartedness

when grounding and "maternal" protection need to be felt, it can be a very nurturing food substance. It may seem odd to receive this quality from an animal food; however, in times of need, it brings us back to our infantlike state of being nurtured, both vibrationally and nutritionally. Small amounts of milk are usually better tolerated. You may want to experiment with different milk sources to see which one supports your grounding vibration best. I have noticed that some people vibrate better to goat or sheep milk than to cow milk. Goat milk imparts a grounding vibration that is forward moving and goal setting, important attributes for someone who lacks self-esteem and direction. Sheep milk adds a sense of the importance of community or tribe to the inherent grounding vibration that is essential for someone who feels isolated or abandoned by family. Cow milk provides a layer of security on to the grounding vibration it creates. Examine your needs and fit them with the best animal energy.

Free-Range Animals, Organically Grown Foods, and Genetically Modified Organisms

The inherent energy of the animal combines with the vibration of the quality of the animal's life. The sum of this vibration is captured within their cellular consciousness. Chickens kept in stuffed compartments fed a predetermined, human-selected feed will have a different vibration than chickens allowed to roam "free range" on a spacious grassy lot. Essentially, we eat our interconnections. If those interconnections are constrained and rigid, this energy will be transferred to us in the eating process. Over the long term, this energy could have quite an impact on our energetic health. Try for yourself as to whether you feel a difference in your energy eating organic, free-range eggs versus conventional eggs!

Similarly, the term "organic" often indicates a more expensive product; however, it also provides us with extra energy currency. When a food is classified as "organic," it means that it was grown by farmers who focus on conserving the soil and water in a way that benefits the ecosystem. Usually, this method of growing implies a natural means, such as not using conventional pesticides, synthetic fertilizers, bioengineering, or ionizing radiation. Organic animal products are from animals that are not given antibiotics or growth hormones. This type of agriculture has a very harmonizing effect on our energy level because it is thoughtful and respectful of the interconnections that come into play in the cultivation of food. In my professional opinion, I tell clients that if it is difficult to afford organic food, select organic purchases carefully. Buy organic animal products whenever possible, as the vibratory quality of the animal may make a greater impact on the human energy field than that of a plant. The animal vibration is closer to that of a human's compared to a plant, suggesting that animal vibrations may be more readily assimilated into human tissue, depending on the health of our root chakra. Therefore, it would behoove us to make the most of what animal foods we eat, especially since most people eat a majority of animal products throughout their life span!

Genetically modified organisms (GMOs) are certainly a threat to our root chakra. GMO foods have a DNA structure that is not natural—it has been synthesized in the laboratory setting. The genes of one plant or animal may have never been combined with the genes of another. We do not know the long-term outcome of these types of combinations, especially with regard to our safety and health. In fact, European countries have banned GMOs from their food supply. Essentially, through human intervention, there is some degree of tampering with the root chakra energy, the DNA, of the plant or animal; therefore, it is only reasonable that consumption of these foods may not be supportive of our root chakra. Eating organic foods is one way to ensure that you are not ingesting GMOs.

Minerals

We know that protein is important for our body and root chakra structures. We eat a large quantity (gram levels) of protein in our diet. There are also micronutrients, or nutrients found in our diet in smaller amounts (1,000 or 1,000,000

Food Allergies

Food allergies, rooted in altered immune function, relate directly to not accessing the powerful protective nature of the Earth. Often, when people with food allergies look at their underlying issues of feeling unsafe, they are able to shift out of having these reactions. Children commonly develop a milk allergy, which is expected to some degree considering they are "new to this world" and are not able to protect themselves. Their ability to ground has not developed to any great extent. It is common that children grow out of these allergies once they have enabled their ability to ground.

Milk-derived products such as cheese and yogurt are important foods for protection. These foods carry the basic grounding nature of animal-derived foods, and they have an added benefit of enhanced protection of the microorganisms used in their manufacture. Most people who are sensitive to milk are not reactive to yogurt, for example, because of the beneficial organisms it contains for the gut. In this way, yogurt is a good food choice for when we feel our defenses are low due to being "unearthed," in a manner of speaking.

times smaller than a gram!), that also impact the physiology governed by our root chakra. For example, calcium is a key root chakra nutrient. About 99 percent of the calcium in our body is stored in the bone and teeth structures. Calcium helps to balance our overall body pH so that our cellular reactions can flow optimally. Foods that supply us with high amounts of calcium (also tend to be high in protein), such as many animal products like yogurt, cheese, and milk, can be very stabilizing to the root chakra. Excessive calcium under certain conditions can lead to the calcification of organs, such as the kidneys. If there is too much energy coming into the root chakra via calcium or protein, this excess could connect to the sacral chakra (located above the root chakra) and influence its function. The sacral chakra governs the kidneys; thus, it is reasonable that they would be affected in root chakra excess.

Iron is another mineral that resonates strongly with the root chakra. It is necessary for healthy red blood cell formation. Much of the more bioavailable iron is present in animal foods like red meat, fish, and poultry, consistent with the ability of these foods to balance the root chakra. However, iron is also found in some vegetable foods such as lentils and beans. Vitamin C works well with iron and, in some cases—such as lemon juice added to a spinach salad—can make the iron more bioavailable from a relatively nonbioavailable source. Another mineral that falls under the activity of the root chakra is zinc. Zinc has a strong reputation as an essential element, as it is needed for thousands of

Vegetarianism

Any reactions to vegetarianism, whether positive or negative, could indicate that there are some issues that require that the grounded vibration be healed. Staunch, righteous vegetarians would most likely be deficient in grounding energy, while adamant, proud meat eaters would be too stuck in their grounded energy, like energetic quicksand or mud. Either way, these individuals are dealing with some issue that belongs, at least in part, to being grounded and safe. Vegetarian diets (at least temporarily) are strongly recommended in individuals with overactive physical, Earth energy. Vegetarian diets, which characteristically have higher levels of complex carbohydrates, will tend to strengthen the higher chakra vibrations.

If an individual would like to balance his ability to ground and be protected, but remain vegetarian, he can do so by eating other foods to balance his root chakra, like root vegetables and legumes. A less physical way is an exercise that involves experiencing the vibration of animal foods through visualization.

reactions in the body involving proteins. Like iron, zinc is primarily found in protein-rich animal foods. Symbolically, calcium, iron, and zinc are all found deep in the layers of the Earth's crust, giving the Earth a strong physical structure. In much the same way, they provide that function to us as human beings, endowing us with a bodily structure and framework that support many of our inner workings to run smoothly.

Interestingly, studies have shown that organic food provides higher levels of minerals (as well as vitamins) compared with conventional food. The matrix of an organically grown food is well supported due to the higher levels of minerals and can confer the same quality to our physical and energetic structures through its high-quality content.

Grounded Imagery Exercise

This visualization focuses on the food or animal image and how the body feels communing with the animal, allowing the energy of the animal to infuse into the feet, legs, bones, and pelvis, finally expressing gratitude to the animal for its contribution of Earth energy. It is important to focus on the integration of the energy with the image. It is not uncommon to feel a warm or tingling sensation in the legs and feet during and at the end of this exercise, as this feeling would denote a renewal of the energy flow between Earth and body.

Close your eyes, put your feet flat on the floor, hands on your legs or knees. Take a couple of deep breaths. Feel your feet connecting with the floor beneath them, feeling the support it provides. See your physical Earth energy moving from the soles of your feet, into the layers of the floor, into the concrete of the building, down through the soil, moving through all layers of the Earth's crust, sinking your Earth energy into the warm, inviting core of the Earth. Now feel invigorating energy from this center traversing back up in the reverse direction, back into your feet, coming up the ankles, the legs, and into the pelvis area. Bring this energy to the sacrum, the base of your spine, and let it sit here for a moment. Note if you see, hear, or feel anything in this space. Allow this part of you to be a safe place, a haven. Trust your impulses from this area. Note any colors, animals, or people in this space. If you sense that you need to balance this center with animal energy, invite a four-legged animal into this sacred, safe place. Ask it to impart to you its high, good, and true qualities that will add to your ability to be grounded, safe, to trust and to be trusted. Allow this quality to flow through in whatever way the animal would like to provide it that you feel comfortable with. Ask that it nourish your physical body in the highest way. At the end of receiving this gift, give thanks to the animal and return to the room by breathing a couple of breaths before opening your eyes.

Root Vegetables

If you could think of just one food that would nourish the root chakra, wouldn't anything that grew deep within the Earth such as a root be a logical candidate? The idea of the root of the body going together with root vegetables is not far-fetched. A personification of the energy of root vegetables is tough, solid, and durable. They are tenacious and determined. After all, they have the large responsibility of linking the entire plant above with the Earth so that it can receive nourishment. They are the ones behind the scenes who are so adept at being focused in their attempt to travel deeper and deeper. In nature's perfectly planned way, root vegetables support deficient or excessive grounded vibrations and all the spiritual issues that go along with them by supplying the organs held by the grounded vibration with the essential nutrients they need.

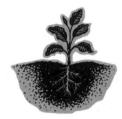

In *Food and Healing,* Annemarie Colbin beautifully exemplifies the essence of root vegetables in the following description:

> Sprouting downward from the seed, the root turns away from the light, burrowing deeper and deeper into the cool, moist Earth. It anchors the upward-growing shoot, drawing nourishment from the soil and sending it toward the sky. It represents stability and strength. Some roots are so powerful that they can crack rocks that stand in the way of their growth.

Root vegetables transfer this grounding energy to the body's collective vibration so that the individual can be firmly planted in who she is and for the purpose of helping her to accept and work with her earthly existence. In our present society, so much emphasis is placed upon the intellect and the upper cavity of the body (for example, brain, face) that the lower cavity and instincts are frequently neglected. Root vegetables, much like the conditions they grow in, help us to nestle into our internal, lower core and to be comfortable in its darkness, quiet, and intuition. In the case of being overgrounded, these foods nourish our feeling of oneness and trust with the Earth and all creation; and for the undergrounded, these foods strengthen the will to exist and to feel supported. Hearty soups made with these vegetables are one example of how they can be incorporated into the diet for nurturing our grounded vibration.

Root vegetables are relatively rich sources of fibers and necessary soil minerals that assist in the structure and function of organs ruled by the grounded vibration. Fiber is symbolic from the standpoint that roots are so tough and durable, making their way into the rocky or soft Earth layers. Tough, insoluble fibers provide us with bulk and solidness, carrying out any foreign material or toxins that get trapped in their network along the way. They enable us to have the sensation of being whole and full of substance, similar to the healthy energy of being grounded.

Aside from fiber, root vegetables supply some essential minerals (selenium, iron, magnesium, potassium) that are crucial for the process of cellular growth and development of structural tissues. For example, magnesium is stored largely in muscle and bones, and it is necessary for muscle relaxation, neuromuscular activity, and protein synthesis, to name a few of its functions. Similarly, potassium is a ubiquitous electrolyte used for a variety of functions, such as muscle contraction and maintenance of cell integrity.

Root Vegetables for Grounding

- Beets
- Burdock
- Carrots
- Celery root
- Daikon
- Garlic
- Ginger root
- Horseradish
- Leek
- Onions
  (red, green, yellow, white)
- Parsnips
- Potatoes
  (gold, red, sweet, white)
- Radish
- Rutabaga
- Shallots
- Taro
- Turnip
- Wasabi
- Yam
- Yucca

Edible and Medicinal Mushrooms

Edible mushrooms such as shiitake, oyster, portabella, button, enoki, chanterelle, morel, and crimini are superb foods for grounding us in our physical bodies. Medicinal mushrooms like maitake, shiitake, and reishi have been explored in traditional medicine systems for their antiviral and immune-enhancing properties. These mushrooms play a helpful role in the body's defense system, in keeping boundaries solid and in keeping the body safe from attack from invaders like viruses. They have a distinct intelligence that resonates with the ancient energy of Earth that keeps us connected to our Earth lineage and physical presence.

Red-Colored Foods

Since the energy of healthy grounding vibrates at a frequency similar to the color red, foods red in color provide the vibrational rate needed to restore our ability to ground. If we are conscious, this vibration can be absorbed visually by both looking at the food and absorbing the vibration as well as by physically consuming the food and incorporating its vibratory rate into our own. This method of repairing our vibration is less effective than eating high-protein animal foods or root vegetables, but it works if we focus our energy on it. Often, people are distracted while eating, to the extent that the appearance of the food is overlooked. Therefore, paying attention to how our food presents itself is therapeutic.

"Red meat" is an example of a food that would be very grounding because of its animal origin, its high protein content, and the color of the flesh. Examples of other red foods include tomatoes, cranberries, raspberries, strawberries, pomegranate, and apples. If someone would ask me what the single most important vegetable food for grounding is, I would answer beets, as they are born within the Earth and they carry the color vibration (red) necessary for grounding.

On a nutritional level, the red plant foods typically provide relatively high levels of vitamin C and plant nutrients referred to as *polyphenols*. These two compounds serve the body in a general sense as antioxidants, or part of cellular and bodily defense. They work to clean up cellular debris and to quench reactive radicals that perpetuate cell damage. Furthermore, they assist the body to protect itself and to establish what is self and not-self. Vitamin C is a potent antioxidant, but it also has several other functions essential to being grounded. Vitamin C helps the collagen matrix form, thereby supporting structures such as bone, teeth, and skin. Vitamin C is also important for the recovery of the adrenals and assisting them to function. Foods high in vitamin C, such as lemons, limes, or grapefruit, would revitalize the root chakra.

Lycopene is one of the plant compounds in red foods that make it red. It is one of the most potent, protective antioxidants and has been shown to be beneficial in the prevention and treatment of cancer and cardiovascular disease. Lycopene appears to be beneficial for reducing risk of prostate cancer. This example indicates how a red, protective compound creates the vibration necessary for healing of the organs in the root chakra such as the prostate gland. If we do not eat red foods, we will be lacking the essential color vibration to keep our root chakra energy fine-tuned.

Red Foods to Feed the Root Chakra

Fruits	Vegetables	Animal Products
Apples (Fuji, Pink Lady, Red Delicious)	Beets	"Red meat" (e.g., beef, buffalo, bison)
Blood orange	Radishes	
Cherries	Red bell peppers	
Cranberries	Red cabbage	
Nectarines	Red chard	
Pink grapefruit	Red jalapeño pepper	
Pomegranate	Red onion	
Raspberries	Red potatoes	
Red currants	Tomato-based products (for example, sun-dried tomato, tomato paste, tomato sauce, salsa)	
Red pears	Tomatoes (for example, vine-ripened, cherry)	
Red plums		
Strawberries		
Watermelon		

AFFIRMATIONS TO HEAL THE ROOT CHAKRA

Affirmations are helpful tools that assist us in changing core belief patterns. By writing these words or by saying them on a daily basis, we infuse our subconscious with new patterns. As we continue to make them a part of our surroundings, so will they become part of who we are. Make up your own as you see appropriate. Here are some to get you started.

- *The core of my being is nourished by foods high in protein.*
- *Root vegetables ground me to the sacred Earth.*
- *Red invigorates me with energizing physical energy.*
- *I give gratitude to the animals and plants that support me with their life-giving presence.*

FOOD AND EATING ACTIVITIES
TO BALANCE THE ROOT CHAKRA

- What belief patterns about food and eating did you inherit from your family? Are these belief patterns still valid for you? If not, list the new belief patterns. List the eating traditions and beliefs you wish to keep. Cultivate these with a fresh start.
- Experience the process of how food is grown. Visit a farm and learn about the farming practices. Buy a package of seeds, plant them in soil. Eat the food that you grow. How is your experience of eating different by doing so?
- Eat close to the Earth, on the ground, barefoot one time per day—write on whether and how this changes your eating experience.
- Note when foods make you feel "grounded" and "ungrounded."
- Practice checking in with your body on food choices. What language does your body use to tell you what and when to eat and when to stop eating?
- Eat a meal that you wouldn't normally eat with your hands with your hands. Have fun!
- Create a community of individuals to eat together based on a shared perspective of food and eating.
- Draw your body on a piece of paper. Ask someone you trust to give you feedback on your drawing—is it accurate? What observations do they note? Set an intention for a healthy body image and for greater acceptance of the gift of your flesh.

EATING PLAN TO SUPPORT GROUNDING

If you are struggling with being grounded and feeling safe, eating foods to support these functions are beneficial. I would suggest that you incorporate grounding foods at every meal so that your daily, earthly existence feels complete.

Breakfast Options
Omelette with red potatoes, spinach, tomato, and cheese
Red Whirl Smoothie*
Cinnamon-Nut Baked Apple*
Morning Scramble*

Lunch Options
Grilled tuna steak in fresh basil sauce served with oven roasted red peppers
Nourishing Bean Soup* with a radish salad
Earthy Chili*
Creamy Cold Tomato Soup* with side of grilled root vegetables

Dinner Options
Garlic chicken with side of curried turnips
Grilled leg of lamb with fingerling potatoes and glazed carrots
Beef tenderloin with grilled onions and broccoli
Winter Root Vegetable Soup* with square of corn bread
Stir-Fried Ginger-Garlic Tofu with Vegetables*
Turkey Loaf*

------

* Indicates recipe at back of book

CHAPTER 5

FOODS FOR FEELINGS AND FLOW

Feeding the Sacral Chakra

*One must still have chaos in oneself
to be able to give birth to a dancing star.*
—FRIEDRICH NIETZSCHE

Water • Creativity • Emotions • Orange •
Sexuality • Relationships • Circle • Polarities •
Pleasure • Movement • Moon • Union

SASHA: ALL SPARKLE BUT NO SUBSTANCE

Sasha adorns herself with bright, colorful clothes. She thrives off the drama occurring at the retail store she works in and fills her spare time watching soap operas. It's easy for her to well up with the events from the day. She feels an incessant need to chat about her experiences with those around her. Her friends see her as a creative, emotional type of person who has many ideas but has not been able to carry them to completion. As a result, she has had many false starts in life. Her list of things to do grows longer each day, and she feels a sense of incompleteness as she is unable actually to achieve something she considers worthwhile. She suffers at some level from being possessed with strong feelings about particular issues. However, her feelings often get the best of her, and she is unable to see out of them to create a solution. She finds herself complaining rather than taking action.

On the surface, Sasha appears extremely friendly, making conversation with those she meets. She involves herself in a number of relationships, although she is unable to truly give attention to any one of them. As a result, they fade quickly. Intimate connections start out very intensely for Sasha but are often ended by her because of her inability to commit emotionally. Finally, Sasha has a history of reoccurring ovarian cysts.

Sasha embodies classical signs of an imbalanced sacral chakra: she is intense, passionate, creative, emotional, friendly, and, on the other side, noncommittal and to some degree superficial. Like Sasha, an individual with an imbalanced sacral chakra might appear as someone who is able to give birth to a multitude of ideas and creative solutions but lacks focus to follow through with any one of them. These are the loud talkers but small doers and achievers. Another manifestation of an imbalanced sacral chakra would be someone who is overly focused on externally achieving without putting in the internal time to flesh out their wellspring of creative ideas. These individuals may capitalize on others' ideas to get ahead but are unable to sustain the creation due to their own inner dearth and insecurity. When their ideas are not implemented, the creative energy they contain can stay within the body energy, creating a physical manifestation involving the most highly creative organs—the reproductive system. Therefore, ovarian cysts could be part of this physiological response. The ovaries symbolize feminine creative potential, and the proliferation and stagnation of ideas become the cyst(s). The end result is that the cyst remains internal, continually growing, until it is extracted. Many cancers are linked to this chakra, particularly cancer of the colon, ovaries, and uterus. Unhealthy sacral chakras become dense and proliferate, creating a condition of compounding dampness. Sasha's healing path includes honoring her creativity and emotions in ways that are beneficial for her body.

THE SACRAL CHAKRA: FLOW

UNHEALTHY SACRAL CHAKRA INDICATIONS

Sasha's situation gives a good overview of someone with a sacral chakra imbalance. If you have issues to address in your sacral chakra, you might answer "Yes" to the following questions:

- Have you been unable to recover from the end of an intimate relationship?
- Are you unable to express emotions?
- Do you often get "weighed down" by your emotions—do they cause you to feel heavy, almost to the point of being immovable in the physical world?
- Do you (*women*) suffer from health issues such as chronic yeast infections, infertility, kidney stones, or endometriosis?
- Have you experienced a traumatic event that you have not been able to recover from and that prevents you from moving forward in your life?
- Do you tend to avoid people because of your discomfort at being unable to fully relate to others?
- Have you given up hope on trying to be successful (whatever that means to you)?
- Are you depressed at your inability to execute on your creative potential?
- Do you feel that you are overly creative, often to the point of exhaustion?
- Do you or have you had cancer, particularly of the colon, ovaries, or uterus?
- Do you often feel that you are moving too fast and that you have nothing to show for your effort?
- Are you fixated on the idea of having something to show for your life?
- Do you often discuss your dreams and wishes with others but are unable to make them happen?
- Are you very successful, but at the expense of others?
- Do you feel that you have a "fear of success" and are unable to implement or deliver what you say you can?
- Do you find yourself in meaningless, random sexual encounters with fear of commitment to anyone in particular?

HEALTHY SACRAL CHAKRA BEHAVIOR

The sacral chakra, nestled in the region of the lower belly, yokes us to the water element and its eternal state of movement and dynamic change. It is the hub of creative potential. Our sacral chakra assists us in wielding and manifesting our internal raw creativity into an external form involving visual arts, body expression, and sound. Artists, painters, musicians, and creators are examples of those in touch with their sacral chakra. When our sacral chakra is functioning optimally, we are able to go with the flow of life and to move as our creative expression calls us, without judgment. This chakra also contains the distillation of the creative capacity of the universe and our ability to harness this energy to manifest our dreams, desires, and passions. Where we put our energy, we will manifest.

The sacral chakra can be perceived as one of movement and dance and likened to the Hindu goddess, Kali, who destroys what is in her path in order to make space for that which is creative and life giving. The people who have been able to live their life's dream, whether making a certain amount of money, raising a family, earning a degree, or attaining cosmic bliss, have a healthy relationship to their sacral chakra. Not only does this chakra delve into the empowerment of the self in terms of its creative expression, it reflects the *relationship* of the self to all living beings in its surroundings—or our relationship with others. Emotions can be the triggers of the creative process within.

A healthy functioning sacral chakra will promote the use of creativity to survive, function, and manifest in this world. An individual who is able to express herself and to be in tune with her emotions and dreams is someone who is in strong communication with her sacral chakra. These people believe that they can exude their uniqueness and still belong and serve the planet with their skills. In fact, they believe that their uniqueness is apparent for good reason: to contribute to the variety, complexity, and creativity of the human race. This individual might present as someone who creates art and shares this expression with others, through the fine arts, graphic arts, cooking, interior design, fashion design, and/or architecture. It could also be, for example, someone who creates a nonprofit organization to benefit environmental issues.

GOING WITH THE FLOW OF CREATIVITY

Our ability to evolve and change our physical form and the environment around us resides within our sacral chakra. In addition to the location of the sacral chakra in the lower belly region, its energy provides the physical groundwork for our being through the ubiquitous presence of water in our cells. Our bodies consist largely of water (60–80 percent), and they respond to the physical shifts and tides of water on this planet. Every hurricane, tsunami, and full moon is felt within the core of our being at the cellular level. As a result, this chakra connects us to the web of those who share the planet with us and helps us to remember the significance of Earth as our "mother"—our "life giver." It is the chakra of sharing with and receiving from others, and realizing that what we do to others, we do to ourselves. The emotions that are felt on the individual level cascade into the feelings of the whole, whether from the level of the cell to the individual or from the individual being to the masses. This center carries the inner and outer dynamics of the evolution of us as a unifed whole to be creative, sensual beings.

The sacral chakra is less dense than the root chakra but is still very physical in its nature. Whereas the root chakra is about grounding to Earth, the sacral chakra is about physical movement outward from a place of internal centeredness. It represents the unformed, but it has all the materials for creation, like a primordial soup or a cosmic dance teeming with chaotic and frenzied emotion, raw creativity, and undulating sensuality.

This chakra speaks to some degree to our ability to "let go and let God." It enables us to surrender to chaos and to dive into a state of absolute surrender or lack of control. The four Laws of Spirit as proposed by Harrison Owen in *The Power of Spirit: How Organizations Transform* represent the release of control in relationship with others that the sacral chakra craves: (1) whoever is present are the right people, (2) whenever it begins is the right time, (3) whatever happens is the only thing that could have happened, and (4) when it's over, it's over. In summary, core issues of emotions, ability to manifest desires, creativity, and evolution of self reside in the sacral chakra.

Core Issues Associated with the Sacral Chakra

- Ability to commit to a relationship
- Ability to express the self and emotions
- Ability to play and have fun, to engage in pleasure and passion
- Acceptance of uniqueness in a diversified whole
- Attitudes toward men and women
- Attitudes toward sexuality
- Implementation of creativity
- Movement of emotions through their cycle

E-MOTIONS

The very nature of emotions is to be "in motion"—hence the symbolism of the spelling, "e-motions." The sacral chakra is the bodily residence of raw emotion. All happiness, sadness, anger, grief, depression, fear, and any combination of these emotions hook in to the gut level of our sacral chakra. If *emotions* relate to an overall experience of a situation, including its perception and interpretation, *feelings* are the response part of that emotional palette. Feelings, the action arm of emotions, are tied to the sacral chakra. The other aspects of the emotion are shared by the higher even-numbered chakras like the heart chakra. Chakras 2 (sacral), 4 (heart), and 6 (third eye) are all keyed into the emotional experience as they provide the energy circuit of the feminine, which embodies emotions, creativity, receptivity, and relationships. The sacral chakra is the pure feeling, whereas the fourth chakra—the heart—works to process those emotions in a compassionate, altruistic way. The sixth chakra—the third eye—processes this emotional input as part of intuition or insight.

Feelings ripple through our physical body. As shown by the research of Dr. Rollin McCraty and colleagues, when we are frustrated, our heart rate and breathing rhythms become jagged and uneven. On the other hand, feeling appreciated results in tandem, synchronous heart and breathing, creating beautiful, consistent waves. It is essential to pay attention to our emotions, since they are an expression of our needs. The more we stifle them, the stronger their call to us. Throughout time, society has downplayed the expression of emotions and emphasized the intellect; however, the two work together for our benefit. Emotions allow us to mine the recesses of our subconscious and ultimately help us to balance our tendency to use the intellect to reason and analyze our external and internal signals.

RELATIONSHIPS

The sacral and root chakras are strongly integrated to provide us with our physical body, instincts, and emotions—the bulk of tools we need to live as human beings on this Earth. The sacral chakra provides us with raw emotions, sexuality, and creative force in physical form to accompany the less physical universal, unconditional love we are capable of (heart chakra). Most important, the sacral chakra is about the energy of relationship in all forms. Merging together the relationship and creative aspects, the sacral chakra holds close to its center issues around sexuality and fertility, spanning the continuum from decisions about childbearing to making choices about sexual partners and even to feelings around sexuality.

Unfortunately, the act of the sexual union has mixed messages in society. Much toxic shame has been generated due to the conflict of what society has told us versus our body's needs. Often, sex is sold as a "lower activity" and accompanied by judgment, which is ironic considering that sexual intercourse is one of the highest expressions of our creative potential as human beings. Essentially, it is the pure exchange of creative energy between two individuals.

The sacral chakra deals with issues of relationship to ourselves and to others in a variety of contexts, including commitment to relationships, being able to cocreate with others, being considerate and respectful of others. In the quote by Sir Arthur Eddington, "We often think that when we have completed our study of one, we know all about two because two is one and one. We forget that we still have to make a study of 'and.'" The focus on the word *and* would represent the sacral chakra. The context in which we form and choose our relationships is the crux of the sacral chakra. This powerful energy center allows us the space to ask ourselves the question: "How do we attract people in our lives to help us learn our message?" Every person we meet is our teacher, and our "enemies" are actually our greatest teachers in disguise.

On a broader and deeper scale, the sacral chakra represents the relationship and unification of universal opposites: yin/yang, anima/animus, male/female, sun/moon, all refer to the double-sided complexity of nature. The sacral chakra contains these dichotomies, allowing them to work together. The shadow side of this chakra resides in conflict between sexes, manifesting as staunch feminism or chauvinism. It may also be reflected as random sexual encounters and the inability to commit to a relationship. Someone who is promiscuous may have conflict residing within their sacral chakra, or perhaps in an effort to be safe (root chakra territory) they overcompensate by putting their sacral chakra in overdrive, which manifests as seeking a number of sexual partners. When there is deficient energy in the sacral chakra, this duality may display itself as indecision or lack of acceptance regarding our feminine or masculine sides. Conversely, there could be balance in the sacral chakra to the extent that both masculine and feminine are able to be held simultaneously in a loving manner throughout our being.

PASSION, PLAY, AND PLEASURE!

Much of our "juiciness" for living life oozes from our primordial, dancing sacral chakra. It holds the sheer pleasure for living and everything that life contains. It is the "fun factor" for our being. Without it, we become stifled, withered, and dessicated. Our life force evaporates. Individuals that have a solar plexus chakra in full gear, manifesting as workaholic tendencies, will suppress the pleasure and play that wants to be expressed by the sacral chakra. The cousin to pleasure and play, passion, needs guidance to evolve into our purpose (carried by the heart chakra), which is the stimulus that gets us to jump out of the bed every morning. Otherwise, misdirected passion can make our lives feel out of control and chaotic. Being able to play shows that we honor the truth of the sacral chakra.

THE NATURE OF THE CREATIVE VIBRATION

A healthy functioning second chakra vibrates to the color orange, which could be perceived as a pure orange or with a tint of red or yellow. Intuitive readings of this chakra may be associated with orange-colored objects like a setting sun or a tiger, or with water symbols like a waterfall, river, or dolphin. Sometimes feminine structures or figures like a mother with child appear in the sacral chakra space. Hidden within can also be images of play, pleasure, and, in women, sexuality. Sometimes the images are not distinct, but are diffuse shapes such as an undulating spiral, which captures the raw energy of this center. The sacral chakra is remarkable for its ability to carry the fertile energy of the planet, spanning from the fiery core to the cool, watery surface.

We have taste receptors in our gut similar to those found on our tongue, so we taste food beyond the mouth, even in the territory of the sacral chakra.

PHYSIOLOGY AND THE SACRAL CHAKRA

The sacral chakra follows our body's hydration status, particularly as it relates to the colon, whose function is to absorb excess water for the formation of stools, and to the kidneys, which are responsible for removing bodily toxins via urine. Also, it oversees the hydration status of every cell of our being and the flow of materials in and out of the cell. Specifically, the sacral chakra symbolizes and governs that which enters and exits the fluid cell membrane. For women, the sacral chakra encompasses the reproductive organs such as the ovaries and uterus. Whereas the root chakra is about a defense strategy of the body, the sacral chakra's function involves an exchange and manifestation of emotions and ideas. Through the vehicle of emotions, this chakra communicates with the other body messengers, like hormones, thereby involving all the chakras of the body. The sacral chakra provides a call to awakening the interconnected nature of the body, and integrating it with the emotions.

Anatomy Associated with the Sacral Chakra

- Bladder
- Hips
- Kidneys
- Large intestine/Colon
- Ovaries
- Uterus

THE RELATIONSHIP OF CREATIVITY
AND FLOW TO FOODS AND EATING

Food and eating represent a functional, survival-based activity; and one of the ways to ensure that we eat is to involve the sensory aspects of our physical body. When we eat, we eat with all of our senses: our sight, touch, taste, smell, and sound. Our physiology and our sacral chakra are designed to ensure that we gain pleasure from our eating experience. There are specific compounds (peptides) released in the gut when we eat a meal that communicate with our brain to help our body decipher that we are experiencing pleasure from the experience. Recently, it has come to light that we have taste receptors in our gut similar to those found on our tongue, so we taste food beyond the mouth, even in the territory of the sacral chakra. Overall, this chakra is strongly and tightly woven into our eating experience at a deep, gut, sensory level, similar to that of the root chakra, although for different reasons. Rather than for pure survival, we look to the food for pleasure with the help of our sacral chakra.

SACRAL CHAKRA FOOD AND EATING HEALING PLAN

Spend Time to Create Meals

In our current culture, we have become dashboard diners, eating in our cars on our way to and from work, shopping, dropping the kids off, or picking them up. A fair number of us live in our cars, which I often refer to as an island or bubble, or are confined to a certain structure of life that stifles our creativity and our ease in preparing meals so that we buy processed foods for the sake of convenience. Due to our busy lifestyles, most people do not take the time to indulge in the satisfaction of creating a meal. Many people admit to me that they do not enjoy cooking and would rather eat out every night. These folks believe that cooking "takes too much time" away from other things; in a time-starved world, cooking is seen by many as excessive. Julie admitted to me that she dreads the cooking process in any form and does not even enjoy eating. It is no surprise that she suffers from ulcerative colitis, a condition that is integrated very closely with the sacral chakra. She misses pleasure in her eating experience.

> This chakra is about relationship—your relationship with others, and with all that is living (including food!).

The sacral chakra gives us the gift of creating a meal, whether it involves hand-selecting items at the grocery store, designing a plateful of food in a colorful way, or even inventing new ways of eating through different silverware or painting your own bowl to eat from. The possibilities of creation through food and eating are truly endless!

Have Everyone Participate in the Creation of the Meal

Taking the time to create a meal for yourself feeds one dimension of your sacral chakra; however, when you create a meal for another, or create a meal with another, the effects on the sacral chakra are magnified manyfold. From the standpoint of nourishing your sacral chakra, eating with others is required. Remember that this chakra is about relationship—your relationship with others, and with all that is living (including food!). I have noticed that more and more people eat alone, usually on the run, not taking much time for it. When we share food with another, our sacral chakra surges with delight—eating becomes pleasurable and purposeful. If you make a meal together, so that two streams of creativity can come together, the sacral chakra regains greater balance. Potluck meals are excellent for this purpose, but meal preparation by a group could extend into the activities before or after the meal, such as setting the table or washing the dishes afterwards. The more everyone's creativity is invested from an energy perspective, the more dynamic the meal experience!

Pay Attention to the Senses When Eating

It is common to eat mindlessly, and even "senselessly"! We can go on autopilot when eating. It becomes an activity to get through rather than be invigorated by. I would strongly recommend really tuning in to the here-and-now when you are selecting, preparing, or eating food so that you can get the most out of your eating experience. Collect yourself into the moment as much as possible so that you can reap the maximum amount of pleasure from the experience. If you are going to eat, why not make the most of it? I like to encourage doing "sensory rotations" by focusing on one sense a week and applying that to your relationship with food and eating. For instance, if you choose taste as your sense, you would be tuned in to savoring the multitude of flavors present in a meal or a snack. Maybe you would put all of your "taste energy" into one food per day, appreciating its flavor with every bite. Now if you are a person with a strong affinity for your sense of sight, you may want to tap into the pleasure of other senses to get their take on eating. You may discover that sight is your favorite sense for taking a nature walk, but that when it comes to food, you receive the most richness from your sense of smell. When you are selecting foods at the market, sample all your senses to ensure that you get a whole palette of experience when you finally sit down to eat!

When we are aware of what we are eating and doing through our senses, we may tend to eat less because our experience of being in touch with our bodies will be much more fulfilling rather than having to stuff down some more bites of food. The pleasure center can become a bottomless pit for endless food if we are not careful. By truly being in the moment of the creation of the food and the eating experience, we maximize our pleasurable interface. And, when our physiology is happy, our psychology reflects this effect.

Engage in Play When You Eat

Your creativity may have been stifled as a child, particularly when it came to food and eating. Do you remember hearing "not to play with your food" as a child? Or to "eat everything on your plate," and often that plate was created for you by someone else without the input of your own choice or creativity? For some families, eating can be a serious and somber event; however, the sacral chakra calls out to transform this tone into one that is fun and light. Rather than seeing eating as a purely obligatory part of your "daily grind," think of how you can turn it into a magical moment of play. When you are eating, sit in the mindset of your childlike self, and play with your food in any way you'd like.

Maybe you create food structures and pyramids as part of your meal designing, or you could use food shapes to dress up the presentation of a meal. One of my favorites is cutting the base off a celery stalk. Looking from the top, it resembles a flower. I can put this art on a serving dish filled with appetizers. Some enjoy food photography to capture the aesthetics and play of food compositions. I have seen food art in which the artist personified fruits and vegetables by giving them faces and even making them appear as animals. Artist Carl Warner has composed amazing "food landscapes" by layering food photos to design a scene.

Eat Foods of All Colors

As part of your sense exploration, the gift of sight can provide so much input. Tune in to the colors of foods. Sometimes when I review what someone has eaten, I refrain from commenting on the actual foods; instead, I focus purely on the colors. Did they get their full rainbow spectrum of healthy, whole foods on this day or that day? A variety of colors in the diet signifies that we are eating rich, whole, complex foods. Let your eyes be tantalized by the colors of food. What draws you in in the garden, or in the market? When you eat foods, take in and savor the array of colors to nourish your aesthetic eye. Not only are the colors beautiful to observe and take in visually, each of them represents an important physiological function that your body is receiving in the eating exchange. Purple compounds like anthocyanidins found in grapes protect the brain and preserve memory function. Orange compounds like beta-carotene found in carrots help maintain vision and a healthy immune system. When you are arranging foods on a plate, think about the foods that fit together in a complementary way. For example, adding diced red pepper or strawberries onto your bed of mixed greens can be very satisfying on both visual and physiological levels.

Eat Foods that Provide a Balance of Tastes

Traditional forms of medicine such as Ayurveda and Chinese medicine encourage the use of all the flavors—sweet, salty, bitter, and sour—in a meal. Research shows that we crave what we do not have in our diet: On high-protein diets, people crave carbohydrates. When we only eat sweet foods, we crave foods that are savory. Therefore, give small amounts of all the flavors to satisfy your tastebuds—both on your tongue and in your gut! Indeed, research shows that we have taste receptors for bitter and sweet in the seat of our sacral chakra territory—in our intestines.

Give Gratitude for the Meal

The sacral chakra is about partnership and exchange. Food provides an exchange of energy, and when we eat, we engage in a partnership with the fruit, vegetables, plants, and animals that have given over their vibration to us. Giving thanks for a meal acknowledges that interchange.

Allow Emotions to Be Expressed

Experts estimate that 75 percent of overeating is due to emotions. In a stressful, busy society such as ours, it becomes difficult to find time to process emotions in a healthy way, such as journaling or exercising. As a means of coping with challenging emotions, people may feel inclined to distract their emotions by eating. Eating offers a temporary quick-fix solution to having to deal with the flow of a feeling. Some feelings are uncomfortable for us to show. For example, it is much less accepted in American society for women to show anger or for men to show sadness. This stigma blocks people from expressing in a way they feel comfortable. When people repeatedly engage in emotional eating, they run the risk of their unfelt feeling accumulating, a process that I call "snowballing." Our emotional baggage builds up and needs to find a release. Engaging in emotional eating only adds to the snowball effect, as it can lead to feelings of guilt. The guilt experienced perpetuates the emotional eating cycle. The best approach for the sacral chakra is to heed the emotional messages it sends forth rather than conjuring up guilt and obsession and having that spill over into the rest of our energy field.

Observe the Symbolism of Food Cravings

The sacral chakra is the seat of magnetism. It attracts what we need into our surroundings so that we can experience and learn. We are drawn to certain foods for a reason. The foods we crave give us pivotal information about our energy state and our emotions. The fact that we are experiencing a craving lets us know that we have feelings that aren't being felt. In the moment of a craving, it would be an excellent practice to do a quick "check-in" with how you are feeling. Are you really craving companionship? Love? Rest and relaxation? Give yourself what you need on a deep level rather than caving

> **Experts estimate that 75 percent of overeating is due to emotions.**

into the superficial indulgence of a craving. If you are unable to access your emotional state and identify what you really need, look at the qualities and inherent symbolism of the food you are craving.

All foods provide messages to us about what we need. Are you craving salty foods like potato chips? Because they connect to unfelt emotions, all cravings resonate with the field of the sacral chakra; however, salty cravings connect with this center more than other cravings. A basic physiological principle is that in the body, water follows salt and salt follows water. Craving salty foods may signal that we have a sacral chakra imbalance that requires us to look at the degree of "flow" in our lives and how much we are allowing ourselves to surrender. Perhaps you find yourself craving sweet foods. These foods provide a mirror to us that we are lacking sweetness and joy in our own lives. Maybe we feel lonely or unappreciated.

What Do Food Cravings Symbolize?

Each food means different things, depending on the individual. However, there are some basic messages provided by certain foods.

Quality of the Food	Ask Yourself:
Salty	Where do you need more flow and openness in your life?
Crunchy	What is stressing you? What feels trampled upon and overwhelming?
Sweet	Do you need more joy and fun in your life?
Spicy	Do you crave intensity and living on the edge? Are you afraid of boredom? Are you bored?
Sour	What do you need to draw your attention to? Do you feel scattered?
Soft	What do you need to sink into to feel comfort? What do you need to do for yourself to feel loved and nurtured?

Give Your Passion Purpose

Of course, there may be cravings that haunt us, and we can do the detective work to uncover their true meanings. Cravings may also be linked to insatiable passion that does not have an outlet. When we direct our passion into our life purpose, cravings fizzle out. In another way, we can connect passion to eating by letting it pour into our experience with foods. I find it interesting that people who are very passionate about life also seem to savor their food to the utmost. When Alan recounts his Saturday evening plans, he delights in describing the minute details of his dinner, including the "zing" of the spices on his tongue from the grilled halibut. He puckers his lips with emphasis when he almost relives eating the blood orange sorbet he made from scratch. When passion infiltrates our lives, it can spill over into our experience with foods and eating to make it that much more "juicy" and inviting!

FOODS FOR CREATIVITY AND FLOW

Foods for creativity and flow often resonate with circular forms. Their vibrational quality is represented by a circle shape, an organic, soft, yielding loop. There is no beginning or end—it is cyclical. These foods assist us in maintaining easiness and pleasure in our lives. Whereas the root chakra imparts a strong, masculine, stabilizing energy, the sacral chakra enforces the need for chaos, union, movement, and feminine energy, and to open ourselves to whatever comes our way.

Water

Foods high in water content, or water intake itself, will support the sacral chakra. It may seem like common sense, but water is one of the most life-giving nutrients we can take in. As Japanese researcher Masaru Emoto, Ph.D., has shown, water is a living entity that is responsive to our intent, thoughts, and emotions. He has shown under a microscope that the crystalline formation of water responds to positive and negative energy. The word *love* written on a glass of water results in well-formed, aesthetically pleasing crystals, whereas placing words like *dislike* or *war* on a container of water leads to broken or fragmented crystals. If we apply these same concepts to our bodies, which are made primarily of water, it would follow that we would be very responsive on the cellular level to our thoughts and emotions.

For the most part, we ingest too little water to support our cellular processes. It is optimal if we can sip water throughout the day, rather than gulping down a glass at a time, in order to keep consistently hydrated. A general rule of thumb is to consume half your body weight in ounces of water, with slightly more in the summer or when you have been sweating profusely. When we are properly hydrated, we are better able to stream with our emotions and our thoughts, and our overall cellular vibration is higher and stronger.

Fats and Oils

A unique property of fats is that they can transform from solid to liquid depending on the temperature they are in. Their dual nature represents the polarity that the sacral chakra embraces. Again, more than any other chakra, the sacral chakra embraces the power of two. The flexible, flowing, and yet static and stabilizing quality of fats and oils make them the best macronutrient for the balance of the sacral chakra.

If we think of fat, we may think of a gel-like yellow glob without realizing that fats are very complex compounds with distinct properties. There are many different families of fats, and each one has its own effect on the sacral chakra. Saturated fatty acids, or more solid, rigid fats found primarily in animal products, give the sacral chakra more structure and support. Many of these fats are of animal origin, so they possess a slightly grounding influence from the root chakra. Saturated fats can harmonize the lower root and sacral chakras so that emotions and creativity can be processed through in a productive, realistic way.

If we zoom in to the level of the cell, we can see that saturated fats can provide some degree of protection to the body since they are incorporated into the border around cells and can prevent substances from easily entering the cell. However, too many saturated fats can lead to too much rigidity within the cell and the sacral chakra. A person eating too many saturated fats may be a "stick in the mud" personality or someone who is not very open to ideas or emotions. These people may be stuck, and, instead of an even layer of protection, the saturated fat may build up within the body, eventually causing unhealthy blocks on physiological and psychological levels. Excessive saturated fat intake has been connected to higher cholesterol and heart issues, which is not surprising considering that the sacral chakra is linked to the heart chakra. If we are unable to deal with the raw emotions generated from the sacral chakra, the heart chakra would be impacted and blocked.

Healthy cell membrane with mixture of fats allowing for adequate flow of substances in and out of cell

Too many rigid saturated fats in the cell membrance leading to less flow

Too many flowing unsaturated fats in the cell membrane leading to too much flow

On the other hand, there are other fats called unsaturated fatty acids. These fats are fluid at room temperature, and they serve a different function physiologically and energetically. These are the fats that are in olive oil, flaxseed oil, and fish oil. Olive oil is a perfect sacral chakra food. It's a core food of the Mediterranean diet. Think of how people in the Mediterranean region like Spain and Italy eat. It's very relaxed and easy, not rushed and rigid. Usually, people in these areas of the world like to eat together, in a group of family or friends, with lots of time conversing and expressing emotions. The community aspect is very strong. Since foods take on the energy of their origin, you can imagine olive oil would reflect many of these qualities. And, indeed, it does. It helps our sacral chakra to express, to enjoy company and sharing, all of which are healthy not only for our sacral chakra but also our heart chakra. You may have heard about how olive oil is heart healthy. It truly is from many aspects.

Now let's shift gears. There are some unsaturated, fluid fats that are not made in our body. The body can make most fats, including saturated fats and the unsaturated fats in olive oil, but not the ones in what is called the omega-3 and omega-6 families. This is the reason we need to include these special "essential fatty acids" in our diet. Essential fatty acids are often more wiggly and mobile relative to other fats, such as the solid saturated fats. They are even more flexible than the fats in olive oil! Like all fats, omega-6 and omega-3 fatty acids are needed as building blocks of the wall around the cell, called the "cell membrane." Without unsaturated, fluid fats, the cell is rigid and does not allow for the easy transport of substances like nutrients and waste products in and out of the cell. Flow is blocked. With the right balance of saturated and unsaturated fats, the cell can release and take in substances, allowing it to function in a healthy manner.

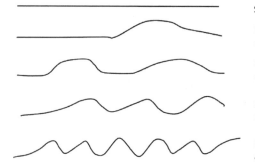

Saturated fat

Monounsaturated fat
(e.g., olive oil)

Polyunsaturated, omega-6 fat
(e.g., corn oil)

Polyunsaturated, omega-3 fat
(e.g., flaxseed oil)

Highly unsaturated, flowing
omega-3 fat (e.g., fish oil)

When the cell does not have a healthy ratio of unsaturated omega-6 and omega-3 fats, it cannot function optimally. If we have too little essential fats, we may get dry skin because the cells in the skin cannot hold water. We may get hair loss and brittle nails. Our body takes on a rigid quality from the inside out. If we have too many saturated fats and not enough essential, unsaturated fats, we may also become more inflamed. We may develop arthritic conditions or heart disease over a prolonged time of not eating essential fats and not allowing our sacral chakra to be nourished and to cool us. In these cases, we have a root chakra excess and a deficiency of the sacral chakra. When we starve ourselves of essential fats, we starve our lower sacral chakra, which leads to a depletion of our higher chakras. For example, a deficiency of omega-3 fats is associated with a number of dysfunctions, including cardiovascular disease (related to the fourth chakra) and mental disorders such as depression (related to the sixth chakra).

Healthy sacral chakra oils include almond oil, butter (due to its animal origin, also resonates with the root chakra), canola oil, coconut oil, ghee (also connects to root chakra), grapeseed oil, olive oil, peanut oil, pumpkin seed oil, rice bran oil, safflower oil, and walnut oil. Two fruits, avocados and olives, could also be part of this list due to the high proportion of healthy oils they each contain.

Fish

The most highly fluid essential fats are commonly found in fish, especially dark, oily fish such as salmon. Salmon is one of the most ideal foods for the sacral chakra since it is a food that lives in the water and is made of these essential, fluid fats. Additionally, its flesh is the color orange, which provides the optimal vibration for the sacral chakra. Other beneficial fish and seafood sources to heal the sacral chakra are anchovies, sea bass, catfish, crab (also resonates with the root chakra), lobster (root chakra), cod, haddock, halibut, perch, oyster, herring, mackerel, menhaden, mussels, orange roughy, pollack, rockfish, sardines, scrod, red snapper, sole, and squid. These fish and sea creatures carry with their physical and energetic structure the essence of life within the flow of water. By ingesting them, we bring these qualities more readily into our nature.

People with a particular aversion to fish may have a "block" or aversion to issues related to their sacral chakra. One aspect to keep in mind is that, due to the high levels of methylmercury found in our current fish supply, it may be advisable to limit fish consumption. Of course, fish containing high levels of methylmercury will not be conducive to the healing of the sacral chakra. The presence of a metal like mercury in fish dams the flow of energy from these fish into our bodies and creates stagnation and toxicity in many aspects of our energetic and therefore physical being. For those who will not eat fish or who want to limit their intake, essential fatty acids of the omega-6 and omega-3 families can be found in much smaller quantities and in various relative ratios in leafy green vegetables, seeds (for example, flaxseed), and nuts. Omega-3 supplements are an excellent alternative and might be warranted for these individuals.

Foods High in Essential Fatty Acids to Balance the Sacral Chakra

- Dark, oily fish, especially salmon, mackerel, tuna; wild is preferable to farmed due to the higher amounts of omega-3 fatty acids in wild fish.
- Flaxseed meal
- Leafy green vegetables
- Walnuts

Seeds

Seeds like flax, poppy, psyllium, pumpkin, hemp, sesame, and sunflower are therapeutic for the sacral chakra due to their rich source of healthy fats. Flaxseed deserves special mention because it is a healing food for the sacral chakra from a couple of perspectives. First of all, it contains oil rich in unsaturated essential fats. Although not as flexible and fluid as the fats found in fish, flaxseed oil can be used in the body to create flow. The other aspect of flaxseed is that it is rich in plant compounds called *lignans*. Lignans act like weak estrogens and are able to compete with estrogen in the body to sit on receptor sites on cells. If the body has too much or too little estrogen, having plant estrogens like flax in the diet could be beneficial. Because of their ability to influence estrogen activity in the body, they are thought to reduce the risk of breast, prostate, and colon cancers. Thus, the energetic and physiological properties of flaxseed fit the needs of the sacral chakra, which oversees the reproductive organs in women and the colon. The benefits can extend into the territory of the neighboring root chakra by protecting against prostate cancer.

Tropical Fruits

When allowed to blossom, the sacral chakra fills and soothes us with delight, joy, relaxation, pleasure, and freedom of choice. It resonates to fruits grown in tropical areas, as they embody these same qualities. Mangoes, pineapple, papaya, banana (also connects to the solar plexus), oranges, kiwi, figs, and coconut are superb examples of nourishing sacral chakra tropical fruits. Eating these fruits enables us to open our inner self to feeling free and relaxed. Coconut and its oil are particularly appropriate for this energetic vibration. Coconut can heal and strengthen the bridge between the two lower chakras. It's a sturdy fruit with a strong protective layer, paralleling the root chakra's boundaries. It is filled with nourishing milk and soft flesh, both which assist the sacral chakra in feeling comfort to open up. Raw coconut butter is a tasty, root-sacral chakra treat!

Nuts

Similar to coconut, all nuts have qualities that strengthen the lower two chakras. The oils in the nuts combined with protein make for a perfect food for combining grounding (root chakra) and flowing (sacral chakra) qualities. Cashews are an excellent choice for the sacral chakra. Note their moonlike structure, resonating with the yin, or feminine quality, of the sacral chakra. Walnuts resemble the complicated brain structure and are, indeed, one of the richest nut sources of omega-3 fats, which are needed for the brain. Almonds, pecans, filberts, hazelnuts, pistachios, Brazil nuts, pine nuts, and macadamia nuts are other fine nut choices to support the sacral and root chakras.

Orange-Colored Foods

As discussed earlier, the healthy sacral chakra vibrates at a frequency similar to the color orange; therefore, viewing or eating orange-colored foods can help to restore the sacral chakra to its correct vibration. Examples of orange foods include carrots, salmon, yams, orange bell peppers, and oranges.

On a nutritional level, most of these orange foods collectively provide beta-carotene (an orange pigment) and other plant carotenoids. Like the red polyphenols used to nourish the root chakra, these compounds are strong antioxidants, but of a different nature than the polyphenols. Specifically, they are absorbed into our bodies with the assistance of fat as a carrier and stored in the cell membranes, similar to the essential fats, where they take on the job of protecting the cell.

Orange Foods to Nourish the Sacral Chakra

Fruits	Vegetables	Animal Products
Apricots	Carrots	Salmon
Blood oranges	Orange bell peppers	
Cantaloupes	Pumpkin	
Kumquats	Sweet potatoes	
Mandarins	Yams	
Mangoes		
Nectarines		
Oranges		
Papayas		
Passion fruit		
Peaches		
Persimmons		
Tangerines		

AFFIRMATIONS TO HEAL THE SACRAL CHAKRA

Affirmations are helpful tools that assist us in changing core belief patterns. By writing these words or by saying them on a daily basis, we infuse our subconscious with new patterns. As we continue to make them a part of our surroundings, so will they become part of who we are. Make up your own as you see appropriate. Here are some to get you started.

- *Water helps my creative expression flow.*
- *My cells are bathed in bliss.*
- *I replenish my inner child with fresh fruits.*
- *Every cell in my body dances to the aliveness of orange foods.*
- *I eat healthy fats that make my cells fluid and flowing.*

FOOD AND EATING ACTIVITIES
TO BALANCE THE SACRAL CHAKRA

- What are your criteria for a healthy relationship with foods and eating? Make an action to become the quality that is first on your list. Write a paragraph on this change.
- Create an affirmation to heal your cravings. Write it down on the left side of a piece of paper and write your immediate response to it on the right side of the paper. Do this five times a day for the entire week. Write about any changes in your craving for the food.
- Make a 2-hour artist's date with yourself this week. Involve food and eating. Write about the experience.
- Make up a funny game to help you deal with a food craving. Play is an important ingredient for the sacral chakra. How can we play with food through games? Create the game and then engage others (speaks to the relationship aspect of the sacral chakra) to play.
- Combine food and creativity in any way you choose, ranging from meal preparation to a unique way to shop at the grocery store (for example, shopping only for green foods) to a novel way to grow food (such as using hydroponics, or the water element, which is conducive to the sacral chakra). Write about your creation and share it with another.
- Invite someone over for dinner and create a meal together.
- Pick an emotion that plagues your daily life and journal on how you better express this emotion throughout your life in a healthy way. How do you "eat" this emotion rather than expressing it? What foods do you gravitate toward when you feel this emotion? What do these foods signify?
- Keep an extensive log of your food intake and emotions. Have one column for foods and another next to it for emotions felt. At the end of a

week, note whether you see any patterns. Do you notice any change in intake when you are feeling more emotional? Are there certain foods you are more attracted to during those times? Or specific foods that you simply cannot eat?

EATING PLAN TO SUPPORT FLOW

It is essential to feel pleasure, play, and passion in your eating experience. As we discussed, your physiology and psychology are intertwined so that you crave pleasure in eating. If you feel stagnant and are lacking fun, eating foods to support the sacral chakra may help you to regain your pleasure center and your ability to feel. Here are some food options to assist you.

Breakfast Options
Honeyed Papaya with Raw Coconut Flakes*
Pleasure Fruit Mix*
Flowing Ginger-Mango Smoothie*
Sprouted grain bagel with smoked salmon and side of cantaloupe

Lunch Options
Carrots dipped in Fresh Almond and Cashew Nut Butter*
Whole grain crackers layered with lox and Walnut Pesto*
Creative Carrot Curry Soup*
Wild Rice-Almond Stuffed Orange Bell Pepper* drizzled with tahini

Dinner Options
Yam Pecan Bake*
Macadamia Nut-Encrusted Halibut* with mango chutney
Grilled Salmon with Apricot Orange Sauce and Baby Carrots*
Mandarin and mango-topped tilapia

---

* Indicates recipe at back of book

CHAPTER 6

FOODS FOR POWER AND TRANSFORMATION

Feeding the Solar Plexus Chakra

I was always looking outside myself for strength and confidence,
but it comes from within. It is there all the time.
—ANNA FREUD

Fire • Inspiration • Presence • Yellow • Accomplishment •
Construction • Triangle • Environment • Self-Esteem •
Will • Dynamic • Masculine • Self-Perception

TOM: ON THE BRINK OF BURNOUT

Tom has a "can-do" attitude and became the CEO of his startup company at age twenty-five, and eventually a self-made millionaire by the age of forty-two. Throughout his life, he has been a rebellious pioneer, exhibiting a strong sense of self-confidence in everything he does and embodying a resist-authority attitude. His nature is to forge through situations fiercely and competitively, with an edge of anger, often leaving others emotionally bruised and battered in his wake. The people that work for him find him at times inspiring, but for the most part overbearing and righteous. He'll give others the impression that he would like to get their input, but truly, he believes that he is the one with the "right" solution. Tom has an outlook on life that could be considered "Machiavellian"— that the end justifies the means. As a result, he never seriously stops to look at his effect on others. In fact, he often thinks that others are too hard on him.

Tom lives a fast life, eating on the run in between meetings or during traveling. Sometimes he even forgets to eat. His digestion has progressively worsened, and he experiences belching and acid in his stomach area after eating. These symptoms do not stop him from his incessant activity, and he continues to push himself to do more. Lately, he has found himself oversleeping on the weekends, feeling so fatigued that he cannot push himself out of bed. But, he analyzes the situation and tells himself he needs to keep going to keep his business profitable. Throughout the years, Tom's weight has been increasing, and recently, his doctor told him that his cholesterol was high and that he is heading in the direction of becoming diabetic. Socially, Tom is quite dominant and intimidating in his relationships with others. He is competitive with his male friends and has a bit of a chauvinistic air about women in general.

Looking on the outside, one might say that Tom appears to be a successful man in that he has wielded his power to become financially secure, have his own business, and be socially active. The underlying question, however, is, What constitutes true success? Does it mean that you use your power to a state of rigid control to get what you want no matter what the price or the effect on others? Tom may be the CEO, but he is not a leader at his core. Rather, he operates from a place of inflated self-esteem and ego so that he can mask the insecurity he feels about his self and abilities. He uses force and competition as the means to get what he wants. His addiction to keep busy prevents him from looking at the real issues in his life that need evaluation. Instead, he busies his mind with excessive analytical and logical thoughts ("analysis paralysis"), squashing his inherent intuitive sense.

Of course, his body has been signaling to him that he is on overdrive and needs to slow down through the excess acid and fatigue that he feels. Tom ignores these signals out of denial that there is a problem, which is symbolic of his approach that he is ultimately calling the shots. His greatest healing would involve removing old patterns and limiting beliefs that no longer serve him so that he can move confidently in the direction that promotes the highest good in him and others.

THE SOLAR PLEXUS CHAKRA: POWER

UNHEALTHY SOLAR PLEXUS CHAKRA INDICATIONS

- Do you feel that you are an overthinker, overanalyzing decisions to the point of exhaustion and confusion?
- Are you fixated on competition and accomplishment?
- Do you feel or have others commented that you are egocentric and self-righteous?
- Are you trying to "do it all," thinking that you have the ability to control all external situations?
- Are you strong in your opinions and unwilling to change or be open to others' views?
- Are you overweight or obese?
- Do you have issues with your digestion such as heartburn or ulcers?
- Are you fatigued from working too hard or too long?
- Do you feel as though you have to overcompensate in social settings due to your lack of self-esteem?
- Are you constantly intellectually stimulating yourself by reading or going to school, but have nothing to show for it?
- Do you feel intellectually exhausted, unable to form any opinions of situations regarding yourself or others?
- Are you reclusive, unable to interact with the external world in any form?
- Do you lack self-esteem and feel that you are going nowhere in life and that you are unable to change?
- Do you feel depressed at your inability to control your life?
- Are you unable to be inspired or to inspire others?
- Do you feel like you lack choices for your life?

HEALTHY SOLAR PLEXUS CHAKRA BEHAVIOR

The solar plexus chakra is conveniently named for its location, which is in the middle of the body trunk, at the level of the diaphragm. Whereas the sacral chakra emphasizes water and understanding our relationship to others, the solar plexus chakra embodies the element of fire and our dynamic, transformative relationship to the external world, encompassing our sense of self, relationship to others, and relationship to our ancestral tribe. It is largely about the self and all of its many aspects: the ego, self-perception, and self-worth. It has the challenging, mammoth task of juggling our inner landscape with that of the outer environment in such a way to allow for harmony and congruence. In fact, in *Anatomy of the Spirit,* Dr. Caroline Myss comments that the solar plexus chakra is the energy center from which we live the most.

Someone with a healthy solar plexus chakra will have the ability to integrate the inner and outer worlds in a way that is effective, productive, and nourishing. There will be a healthy exchange of energy flow from this center outward and coming inward. The ability to integrate environments is rooted in a strong foundation of belief in oneself and proper balance of perception relating to others. These individuals are able to live authentically, as who they truly are, without the burden of a mask. A healthy solar plexus chakra will lead to a feeling of accepting the perfection of our imperfections. At this level, there is comfort with knowing who we are and taking it all in without judgment. In addition to accepting their inner worlds, individuals with healthy solar plexus chakras are able to put the input from the world, whether from news events or from a word spoken by a colleague at work, into perspective without diminution or inflation. They will not be prone to obsessing over a comment about their appearance or gloss over constructive feedback from a mentor. As a result, the outer world will not feel overwhelming to them.

These people are often very balanced, and you can spot them by their ability to do many things in life at once, such as have a family, career, and social life with ease and grace. Somehow, the elements of their lives synchronize in a way that gives them a sense of calm and control rather than deplete them of energy to the extent that they are perpetually fatigued.

The area governed by the solar plexus is essentially our seat of "power." It is the gateway to the reaping in and the dissemination of energy in our lives. This chakra provides "fuel" for our self's expression—this center is able to transform and harness the energy we take in from the outside for all the internal layers of the self. Its mission is to direct our energy outward in ways that reflect our self-esteem and self-worth. In its highest state, it reflects the pure brilliance and the light of who we are shining forth to all. A healthy solar plexus chakra will be reflected in an individual who is radiating inspiration, dedication, and motivation just by entering a room. These individuals embody what cultural anthropologist Angeles Arrien, Ph.D., refers to as the power of "presence." They command respect not through the aggressiveness of their words but through their actions to

Core Issues Associated with the Solar Plexus Chakra

- Ability to express the self and its needs
- Ability to manifest personal power in the world
- Attitudes toward the self
- Feeling a sense of control regarding life outcomes
- Filtering perceptions from the external world and determining how they fit within the belief system of the self
- Forming an opinion
- Thinking logically

empower others. Power is gained not through demeaning others but by uplifting and inspiring them in a way that leads them to find their own brilliant self.

MANIFESTATION

The solar plexus chakra is the last of the chakras of what we might call a "physical" nature; it is the highest of all the physical body chakras. It delivers on the mission of the root and sacral chakras through the act of will. With the assistance of the solar plexus chakra, the dreams and creativity harbored in the sacral chakra can be made externally manifest. It contains the ability to take raw, swirling chaos and desire and turn it into conscious, linear beams of light and purpose. The masculine energy of the solar plexus puts action together with the creative force, leading to the creation of a future strung together by pearls of goals and achievement. The solar plexus chakra takes us forward in the direction of our dreams with the internal knowingness that there is the capacity to succeed. Furthermore, the achievement of our dreams is accomplished through a dynamic interaction between our internal wellspring of knowledge, talent, and belief, coupled with that of external group efforts.

IDENTITY

The solar plexus region at the center of the body is symbolic of the link between the upper ("heaven") and lower ("earth") parts of a being. It is the doorway between the self and the rest of the world. Imagine it as a netted filter. Some of us have larger openings in our filter and therefore allow much to go out and to come in. Others have smaller openings in their filter, allowing only select pieces to come in and out. This filter is a place of collection and entry of that which flutters around our being in the external world—it can collect whatever we allow it to, including any thoughts, criticisms, perceptions, opinions, stereotypes, judgments, and so on. If we do not protect this center adequately, we are left open to the energy thought forms that are around us, generated by mass consciousness, whether or not we choose.

Because of the filterlike nature of the solar plexus chakra, it is essential to keep the energy moving within it, perhaps slightly more than the other chakras. This chakra responds quickly to the external climate on many levels. It can take in and integrate the consciousness of a group of friends we are sitting with, or the state of the world at large, and even the effects of monumental physical vibratory shifts in the Earth. Large-scale issues that affect humanity, such as wars, can greatly impact the solar plexus chakra energy.

The solar plexus center starts to evolve around the time we start to create our identity, which is usually from seven to ten years old, and it can collect perceptions about us passed down by our parents. It can be molded and shaped according to these perceptions, setting a template for the adult self. As we become adults and find ourselves in repeated negative predicaments, it may be worthwhile to get a closer glimpse of this area to see what limiting beliefs we have stored within this center. We could be creating a wall with the exterior, which could lead to isolation, or we may be too utterly giving, without firm boundaries on our thoughts and beliefs, resulting in exhaustion. Often, as we shed our identity formed as a child and morph it into a new adult identity, our solar plexus chakra may generate feelings of duality—foundational beliefs confronted with new ways of thinking and feeling. Traits of indecisiveness and combativeness are hints that this process is occurring. This period is what is known to astrologers as the "Saturn return." We usually emerge from this process with a tweaked set of beliefs, values, and opinions.

> **Because of the filterlike nature of the solar plexus chakra, it is essential to keep the energy moving within it.**

THE MOST IMBALANCED CHAKRA?

Most people in the Western world appear to have issues residing in their solar plexus chakra more than in any other chakra. Through my own research using the questionnaire in this book, I have found that up to 80 percent of North Americans and Europeans tested have a predominant solar plexus chakra imbalance. Why is this? Actually, this finding may come as no surprise to many of you. We live in a power-hungry, stress-filled society that is always expecting more and more of us. Our ability to maintain balance in the midst of chaos becomes increasingly difficult when demands and responsibilities begin to pile high. We try to accommodate by saying "Yes" when we really mean "No," and after awhile, we feel burdened with life and everyday events become drudgery. Finally, we collapse in a state of exhaustion.

On the whole, our solar plexus chakra, and ultimately, our entire being, is responding to this current era of excess. We are living in an age of an incredible amount of energy transfer at faster and faster speeds. We have the Internet, email, and wireless handheld devices so we can soak in every particle of the constant stream of energy available to us. When there is an excessive amount of energy being taken in, there may be an inability to integrate this energy with the self. Often, this imbalance manifests as weight gain in the abdomen, particularly when the individual takes in energy and cannot balance the intake with the output. Weight gain can also be seen throughout the body as a way of "protecting" it from the outside, for whatever reasons. The nationwide obesity epidemic is due in part to the huge amount of energy coming in (high stimuli, increased workload, busy schedules) and a depletion of internal energy resources. For example, Sam came into the clinic complaining of persistent weight gain. Looking closer, it was revealed that he was going through a divorce, had a major job change, and his daughter was having problems in school. He was barely able to sleep a solid three hours a night! Most times, he would forget to eat or eat convenience foods late at night once the kids were in bed. He was experiencing severe internal energy depletion—he was doing nothing in his life to nourish him. Once he started eating more regularly and eating certain foods, he was better able to concentrate at his new job and sleep six hours a night. He began losing weight

> **Most people in the Western world appear to have issues residing in their solar plexus chakra more than in any other chakra.**

slowly over the weeks. Four months later, he decided to run a marathon, like he had done fifteen years ago—he now had the energy to give out.

Conversely, too much energy given out and an inability to take energy in can lead to a host of different conditions. This situation is often seen with over-achievers, or working single mothers, who can easily overextend themselves by working, going to school, and trying to raise their children on a compromised income. The end result is pure fatigue from an overdrive of energy being given out of the solar plexus chakra. After awhile, the body is depleted of physical, mental, and emotional power, and chronic disease results, particularly centered in the area of the digestive organs. For example, our stomach can lose its ability to break down and transform foods we eat. The end result is the fermentation of undigested food in the stomach, subsequent acid reflux, and even ulcers.

The solar plexus chakra is our energy account. Take a look at your energy flow. At any given moment of time, we have a certain amount of energy. Some people put their energy in the past, some in the future, some in both the past and future, and as a result have no energy to live in the present. The solar plexus chakra is our measure of overall energy, or *chi*. When we feel drained, we need to be careful about how we are delegating our internal resources. Are certain external environments leaving us dry? Do other activities give us energy in return?

THE NATURE OF THE POWER VIBRATION

In its highest form, this center vibrates to the yellow and gold colors of the sun rays. Intuitive readings of this chakra may be associated with the color yellow or yellow objects, such as a sun, sunlight, or a lemon. It is also associated with more masculine structures and objects of organization, such as builders, con-struction, and ladders. Sometimes there is a hint of fire or even metal images.

PHYSIOLOGY AND THE SOLAR PLEXUS CHAKRA

The solar plexus center is connected to the organs in the body responsible for transformative processes, namely the digestive system, encompassing the esophagus, stomach, pancreas, small intestines, liver, and gallbladder. It is the hub of our physical relationship with food and represents the exchange of infor-mation with food and our body's ability to decode the information into signals. The nutrients signal a transformation throughout our body known as metabolism, the sum of building and breakdown reactions. On a cellular level, this center is linked to our mitochondria, or our cellular powerhouses, whose job it is to extract the raw energy from starting materials supplied by foods. This chakra is strongly linked to both the first (root) and fifth (throat) chakra. Together, this network symbolizes the ingestion (fifth/throat chakra), digestion (third/solar plexus chakra), and elimination (first/root chakra) of food. Furthermore, the throat chakra, as you will read in chapter 8, is responsible for thyroid function and other hormones. These hormones work with the digestive organs to control appetite and metabolism.

Anatomy Associated with the Solar Plexus Chakra
* Gallbladder
* Liver
* Pancreas
* Small intestine
* Stomach

On a physical level, people with well-functioning third chakras tend to have robust digestion and metabolism, and they are often of medium build and average weight. These people are the ones who can "eat almost anything" and get away with it. They tend to be able to digest relatively large portions of food in one sitting. Also, people with healthy third chakras tend to have energy endurance; they are usually physically and mentally active.

THE RELATIONSHIP OF POWER AND TRANSFORMATION TO FOOD AND EATING

Food represents energy on many levels, spanning from physical to spiritual. All of these energies feed us with the power we need to make our way in the world, whether taking a step, uttering a word, or thinking a thought. Our bodies are beautifully equipped with the necessary organs to transform the energy of foods into an energy that we are able to use, similar to what a language interpreter would do. The solar plexus chakra is the hub of this transformation: it provides a centralized location for the digestion and absorption of the foods we eat. No other chakra contains the degree of specialized function for liberating energy like the solar plexus chakra. The food we eat transforms us. If it carries energy that is nourishing, we become nourished. If it harbors the energy of anger, we take on that anger. Thus, this center is the key for unlocking the messages of food.

SOLAR PLEXUS CHAKRA FOOD AND EATING HEALING PLAN

Know When You Are Hungry

Power signifies a strong current of energy. When we are empowered, matter (our bodies) connects with movement (action) to give us direction and focus. When we are able to fuel our bodies appropriately, they can receive the food messages with clarity, helping us to concentrate on tasks at hand. Many individuals have lost their way in reading their bodies to know whether or not their fuel (food) gauge is empty or full. When we overeat, we overwhelm our organs of transformation. Our stomach takes on an uncomfortable feeling as it is unable to process the food that has emptied into it. It remains bloated and acidic, releasing undigested food into the small intestine for further digestion. The small intestine is not always equipped to digest excess food. It may not be able to produce enough enzymes to break down the starches. The liver may not be able to produce enough bile to solubilize the fats we take in.

By overeating, we impair our body's ability to transform the foods into energy. We may even become drained of energy in the process. Think of any number of Thanksgiving dinners you may have participated in, when you felt heavy and lethargic after eating. We can tax our transformative power by excess input of any form, including foods.

On the other hand, undereating will lead to a deficit in energy. We will rob our system's resources since not enough of them are coming in. When we do not eat, we can become low on energy, similar to the same effect as overeating. Only this time, we are low due to the lack of energy "funds." Under these circumstances, we also find it difficult to concentrate. The liberation of quick-energy glucose from foods helps our brain to function better. When we lack foods, we starve our concentration potential.

It is best to retrain ourselves to be in touch with senses of physical hunger. Note when hunger originates from your gut area (solar plexus) rather than when you are simply "thinking about" being hungry. Is your stomach rumbling?

Do you feel an empty pit in that area? If you do, your body is asking you to pay attention and to fill it with fuel, with energy, with power so that you can live a transformative life. This is a signal from your solar plexus chakra that you have put out too much energy and need to take some in again to replenish your stores. And when you eat, don't saturate your system. Various sources have commented that an optimal intake is having a sensation of being 80 percent full. My recommendation is that you eat just enough so that after eating you can move comfortably around, such as taking a light walk. Make sure that you aren't tired after eating, as that can be a sign that you have eaten too much!

Exercise: Know Yourself, Rate Your Hunger

It is useful to journal on your food intake and to rate your hunger after a meal. Use a 1–6 scale (see sample below), with "1" being "ate just enough" and "6" being "painfully full." Doing this activity will assist you in becoming more conscious of your food intake and allow you to exercise your ability to sense your body's signals of hunger and fullness. Of course, being aware of physical hunger and satiety (feeling of fullness) is important, and essential for tuning in to your body's wisdom about foods and eating. When you are hungry, your energy reserves are low. By paying attention to your solar plexus chakra and your eating times, you will be better suited to deal with the stresses of everyday life. Each time you complete this exercise ask yourself whether you are surprised by your ratings. See whether it becomes progressively easier to connect with your internal signals from your solar plexus chakra.

Sample Scale:
1. Ate just enough
2. Ate slightly more than I should have
3. Went past my limit, and feel "full"
4. Ate excessively, too full to think about
5. Uncomfortably full, feelings of regret
6. Painfully full, unable to move, feelings of guilt and disappointment

Be Aware of Food Energy

Similar to either overeating or undereating, we may be eating foods that either give us optimal energy or that take our energy from us. Have you ever had the experience of eating a small portion of a specific food and after eating it felt like it wiped you out? And, you may react differently to foods at various times of the day or at random periods of your life. These foods will be different for everyone. It is up to you to be aware of your body and spirit reactions. Anna comments, "Every time I drank orange juice, it was like crushed glass in my stomach." Even though most people may enjoy, crave, and need orange juice, there may be some individuals who react adversely to its ingestion. Usually, we get a quick, definite reaction from our solar plexus region as to whether or not a certain food suits us within a couple of bites.

Another example is Rob, who struggled with his addiction to caffeine. Throughout the day, he felt pulled to saturate himself with highly caffeinated beverages, starting with several cups of dark coffee in the morning and a few soft drinks in the afternoon. Sometimes he'd drink a canned "energy drink" in the evening if he had plans to go out. One day he skipped his morning caffeine routine and became fatigued and nonproductive by early afternoon. He felt like a zombie, completely lifeless and devoid of his drive. Looking deeper within, he came to the realization that caffeine had him in its grip and that much of his energy was determined by his caffeine intake. Rather than allow himself to be fueled by this substance, he decided to take his power back by cutting down his intake, getting to bed earlier, and taking short brisk walks throughout the day to reenergize. He also replaced his sugary snacks with tasty, high glycemic foods like a trail mix made of nuts and seeds.

If we couple eating the foods that cost us energy with overeating, we are really looking at a severe taxing of the solar plexus chakra-organ interface. Karin told of how she was in bed for days after having a large Mexican food lunch with wheat tortillas. She knew that she didn't do well with wheat, yet she proceeded to eat a number of flour tortillas. Of course, she learned that this combination led to severe imbalance. On the other hand, some foods may impart a burst of energy. Sue states, "Every time I eat steamed broccoli, I feel full of good, healthy energy. It's like fuel for me to function better."

Schedule Regular, Frequent Mealtimes to Prevent Energy Loss

The best strategy for ensuring a steady quantity of energy throughout the day is to eat small, frequent meals five to six times daily. You may have heard this recommendation for diabetics, who need to keep watch on their blood sugar levels. When we eat small portions throughout the day, we are able to digest them better. Furthermore, we are able to keep our blood sugar levels steady rather than creating sharp blood sugar peaks and drops that cause us to feel unstable, lightheaded, and fatigued. Feeding the solar plexus chakra regularly will ensure that you have the proper amount of fuel to keep you feeling charged throughout your day.

There are times in the day when we are better able to digest than others. For example, in traditional medicine systems like Ayurveda, noon is the hour when the metabolic fire burns brightest. It is at this time that the transformative action of the solar plexus chakra is blazing, much like the sun at its highest point of the day. Conversely, late at night is when our transformative potential is at its nadir. We are unable to efficiently process food in a way that is energizing. It often takes some degree of un-training for people to reverse their pattern of eating heavy dinner meals, but the body does adapt quickly if we are open to it.

Balance "Warming" and "Cooling" Foods

The solar plexus chakra is all about fire and heat. It is with the element of fire that alchemy takes place. Metals can become soft and pliable in the presence of fire. Cooking food changes its structure, which then changes its digestibility. Fire purifies and cleanses. The act of eating is transformative in a way that is cleansing to the body. It renews and invigorates the body. When we eat raw food, it requires our solar plexus chakra to work harder to tear down the strong natural bonds present in plant foods. When we cook food, the structure changes so that it is often easier to digest and absorb. In traditional Chinese medicine, raw foods are often contraindicated for people who over-think (spleen *chi* deficiency).

From a chakra perspective, this idea makes good sense. If you are an over-thinker, you may be depleting your solar plexus chakra by putting out too much "thought" energy. Eating raw foods will only cause you to have to expend more solar plexus chakra energy. Therefore, cooked foods may be better suited in this condition. On the other hand, for someone with too much solar plexus energy, such as high-energy, on-the-brink-of-burnout Tom, having some raw foods may be beneficial because they can help to dispel some of the pent-up solar plexus energy, thus having a "cooling effect."

The lower three chakras resonate to the three main energy-providing nutrients: the root chakra builds its foundation with protein, the sacral chakra flows with fats, and the solar plexus chakra liberates energy from carbohydrates.

The other type of "hot food" is food that is spicy. In certain restaurants, you may be asked how spicy you would like your food to be and even give a number on a scale to grade the intensity of spiciness. Spices like black pepper speed up the digestion and absorption processes and rev up the solar plexus chakra. It can cause a feeling of heat in the body, causing sweating. It provides a warm, internal flood of energy to invigorate the solar plexus chakra. In my experience, it seems that people who enjoy spicy food crave intensity and warmth in their lives. Their solar plexus chakra may not be taking in enough excitement, and they can provide this quality through spicy food.

FOODS FOR POWER AND TRANSFORMATION

Foods for power and transformation are symbolized by the triangle. The triangle represents a base with clear direction and focus, indicated by the pointed top. The triangle also symbolizes the number three, or the culmination of the root, sacral, and solar plexus chakras. The solar plexus is like the "father" of the lower chakras, taking in all the energies and directing them outward to interact. In much the same way, foods that create sustained energy are represented by the triangle nature.

Carbohydrates

The lower three chakras resonate to the three main energy-providing nutrients: the root chakra builds its foundation with protein, the sacral chakra flows with fats, and the solar plexus chakra liberates energy from carbohydrates. Carbohydrates are able to provide the solar plexus chakra with what it needs: everything from quick energy sources like glucose to long-lasting sugar sources like fiber.

CARBOHYDRATE QUALITY

There are all different types of carbohydrates, ranging from simple sugars to complex starches. If the solar plexus chakra requires a slow release of energy to accommodate for a consistent output of energy, it would be best served by carbohydrates that slowly release sugar (glucose) to the bloodstream. These carbohydrates are often referred to as "low glycemic index" carbohydrates. Some carbohydrates have a particular structure that takes longer for the body to break down. Often, but not always, low glycemic index carbohydrates are those carbohydrates referred to as "complex." For example, brown rice is both a low glycemic index and complex carbohydrate. On the other hand, an apple may be considered as a quick energy source, since it consists of simple sugars. However, the sugar it contains is primarily fructose, which has a low glycemic impact.

To understand the glycemic index concept further, think of sugar entering your bloodstream like water coming out of a faucet. If you turn on the faucet all the way, so that the water is rapidly streaming out, you may fill up the sink quickly. It may even overflow. In much the same way, when we eat foods that have a high glycemic index, the simple sugars from the food quickly appear in the blood and we get high blood sugar. Conversely, when we eat low glycemic index foods, it is like letting the faucet dribble out water every couple of seconds. In this scenario, these foods slowly release glucose into the blood. Foods that have a low glycemic index, like grains, beans, and vegetables, would be nourishing to the solar plexus chakra. Foods that have a high glycemic index are those that are "quick-fix," high-energy foods that deplete the solar plexus chakra, like the following:

- High-sugar desserts such as cakes, cookies, donuts, ice cream, candies
- Starchy snack foods such as crackers, potato chips, tortilla chips
- Starchy vegetables such as corn and white potatoes
- Fruit juices with added sugar
- Processed breakfast cereals
- White rice
- White bread products such as bagels, muffins, sliced bread

What the science has shown us is that eating low glycemic index foods results in a panorama of health benefits, including improved body weight, blood lipids, blood sugar and insulin, and better appetite control. Rather than being out of control with our hunger cues, and even having our appetite control us, we are able to keep a better rein on our hunger when we eat foods that give energy to the solar plexus chakra.

Healthy Low Glycemic Foods to Sustain the Solar Plexus

Legumes	Vegetables	Whole grains
Bean soups	Broccoli	Barley
Canned or cooked beans (garbanzo, soybean, black, pinto, lentil, etc.)	Cauliflower	High-fiber wheat tortillas
Hummus	Dark green leafy vegetables (spinach, kale, dandelion greens, collard greens)	Oatmeal (whole rolled oats, steel-cut oats)
	Green peas	
	Tomatoes	
Nuts	**Fruits**	
Almonds, hazelnuts, walnuts	Apples	
Hazelnuts	Berries	
Walnuts	Cherries	
Nut butters (unsweetened)	Grapefruit	
	Pears	

CARBOHYDRATE QUANTITY

Another point to consider is not only the quality of carbohydrate, but the quantity of carbohydrate relative to the other macronutrients such as protein and fat. There always seems to be an ensuing debate about what level of carbohydrate in the diet is best. High-carbohydrate diets, such as those exceeding 60 percent of the total energy from carbohydrate, could lead to an overworked solar plexus chakra, whereas extremely low-carbohydrate diets, such as those in the range of 20–30 percent of the total energy from carbohydrate will result in less energy expended by the solar plexus chakra. One may have to modify the carbohydrate level of his diet depending on the state of his solar plexus chakra.

The high-protein, low-carbohydrate craze cycles through the popular literature fairly regularly. As we discussed in chapter 4 on the root chakra, this trend mirrors our need for more grounding due to the high protein. It also indicates the need to reserve the energy going through our solar plexus chakra so that we do not become depleted.

Fiber

Specifically, fiber refers to the part of a plant that is not able to be digested. On a basic level, there are two types of fiber: soluble and insoluble. Insoluble fibers are the nondigestible carbohydrates that go through our digestive tract relatively unchanged. They are usually referred to as being "broomlike" in that their structure moves through the long tunnel of intestines, carrying other bulk in the intestine through with it until the end. These fibers are for moving digested food and other secretions through the intestine. They support the activity of the lower chakras, especially that of the sacral and root chakras in that they provide movement and flow of bulk (sacral chakra) and they are found in the outer skins of fruits, vegetables, grains, nuts, and beans, indicating that they serve as protection (root chakra).

The other type of fibers, called soluble fibers, sustains the solar plexus chakra and also plays a role in maintaining balance in the sacral chakra. They are found underneath the insoluble fiber sheath of plants. For example, an apple contains insoluble fiber in the red skin, and soluble fiber in the whitish flesh of the apple. Soluble fibers have a structure enabling them to swell in the presence of fluid. They become viscous and gel-like and are able to form a matrix to trap particles like sugars so that they are released slowly into the bloodstream. This extended release assists the solar plexus chakra in harnessing its energy input. These fibers are also called "prebiotics" because they can also be fermented by the bacteria in the gut into healthy short-chain fats that have a variety of health functions, including stabilizing blood sugar.

Unfortunately, most Americans fall short on fiber. It would be interesting to note whether we might have fewer solar plexus chakra issues if we were eating more fiber in our diets. It is important to eat high-fiber foods when we are engaged in strong mental or physical activity, such as a sports competition or even working at the office. These foods prevent the injury of the glucose sharp spike in the blood and plummeting dip within hours. High-fiber foods are able to sustain the release of glucose into the blood for constant energy. In turn, the solar plexus chakra is able to be fed and supported when the mind and body are overextended.

Food Sources of Insoluble and Soluble Fiber
to Balance the Lower Chakras

Insoluble Fiber	Soluble Fiber
Fruits	Flaxseed meal
Nuts and seeds	Fruit and fruit juices (tomato, plum, berries)
Vegetables (carrots, cucumbers, zucchini)	Legumes (dried peas, lentils)
Wheat bran	Psyllium seed husk
Whole grain foods	Vegetables
Whole grains (oats, rye, barley)	

Quick-Release Sugars

Foods that would block or imbalance the solar plexus chakra include those that release quick, rapid energy due to the exceptionally high content of simple sugars, such as cookies, soft drinks, and candy. These foods tend to be processed and refined, and not whole and complex. Orange juice will react differently in the body compared with eating an orange. The juice, made from the collection of simple sugars from more than one orange, will be high in simple sugars and give a quick burst of energy to the solar plexus chakra. In contrast, when you eat an orange, it slowly releases the natural sugars from the matrix of the fruit into the body.

Foods high in simple sugars cause much energy to enter the body's energy rapidly without a compensatory constant output. In fact, much of the body's energetic reserves are utilized to balance the body after ingestion of these foods. Have you ever noticed how tired you might feel an hour after having a sugary snack? Initially, the burst of energy coming in may feel energizing, but as our body processes the sugars quickly, we are left in a "sugarless" state. We feel used up and tired. We may even get into a cycle of reaching for another sugary snack to invigorate our solar plexus chakra once again. This cycle causes our solar plexus chakra to be depleted of any energy coming in to this center. An easy indicator that someone has issues in their solar plexus chakra is that he will crave quick-fix carbohydrates such as pretzels or cookies. If the pattern continues, and it is coupled with erratic eating patterns like eating too often or not frequently enough, he will throw off his careful metabolic balance and set himself up for conditions like obesity, metabolic syndrome, and subsequent development of diabetes.

Sweeteners

In many ways, we are a society addicted to sugars. When we eat high-intensity artificial sweeteners and processed sweeteners like high fructose corn syrup, our body's baseline for sweetness reaches an unnatural state. After a certain time, it is difficult to find anything like natural sugars or fruits satisfying because of the high taste expectation we have created. The real question is, Why are we craving such high-intensity sweetness? What sweetness are we missing in our lives? What is out of balance? As you may recognize, people who are burdened with stress and responsibilities have burnt up the energy in their solar plexus chakra. Their natural reaction is to look for sweetness in their food to give them the temporary sensation of energy and delight. However, by doing so, we are setting ourselves up to drain ourselves further of energy.

> An easy indicator that someone has issues in their solar plexus chakra is that he will crave quick-fix carbohydrates such as pretzels or cookies.

High-Intensity and Balanced Sweeteners

High-intensity sweeteners are disguised in many forms. Here are some names of natural and artificial sweeteners to look for on labels and stay away from: sucrose, high fructose corn syrup, evaporated cane juice, honey, raw sugar, turbinado sugar, brown sugar, confectioner's sugar, powdered sugar, dextrose, glucose, molasses, corn syrup, maltose, saccharin, aspartame, Equal, NutraSweet, sucralose (Splenda), and acesulfame potassium. Sweeteners that are more balanced (and have a low glycemic index) are agave nectar, apple juice concentrate, and stevia.

When we let go of unnatural sweeteners, we similarly open space in our lives for the natural flow of sweetness to enter and for our solar plexus chakra to be balanced and free.

Jane is a perfect example of someone who was trapped by high-intensity sweeteners. She would start her morning with a sweetened cold cereal and white flour bagel with honey. On her way to work, she would stop for an iced latte. By ten in the morning, she already felt like her energy was dragging and that she could not focus on her work. She would eat some candy to help her pick up her pace, which helped initially, but then she quickly found herself back to where she started. By mid-afternoon, she was so sleepy that she would have at least one soft drink to give her some caffeine. It is no wonder that she would come home in the evening so exhausted that she couldn't make dinner or go to the gym to exercise. Many people have their days unfold like Jane's.

A quick burst of sugar in the morning followed by more and more sugar to the point where they become overrun with fatigue. Once Jane eliminated all sources of processed sweeteners in her diet, she realized that her sugar cravings had stopped entirely within ten days. Her tastebuds started to get used to the sweetness of whole fruit and of healthy, natural sweeteners like agave nectar and stevia. Her fatigue dissipated and she was able to function better in her job. Changing her diet helped her to focus on more sweetness in her life such as taking an evening class on watercolor painting. Her solar plexus chakra was brought back into balance!

> **When we eat high-intensity artificial sweeteners and processed sweeteners like high fructose corn syrup, our body's baseline for sweetness reaches an unnatural state.**

Legumes

Legumes provide a balanced source of both protein and carbohydrate. They are key foods for aligning the root and solar plexus chakras. The protein provides a means of grounding, while the complex carbohydrates they contain allow them to trickle in energy slowly to support the solar plexus chakra. As a result, they impart a slightly heavy, filling feeling when we eat them. I recommend that individuals get at least $1/2$ cup of legumes daily to help balance their lower chakras. All legumes are useful, including orange/green/brown lentils, garbanzo (chickpea) beans (includes hummus), butter beans, black-eyed beans, navy beans, cannellini beans, fava beans, pinto beans, green beans, kidney beans, black beans, lima beans, white beans, soybeans (could be dry roasted or fresh edamame), fat-free refried beans, adzuki beans, mung beans. A creative recipe using beans is provided in the solar plexus chakra recipe section at the end of the book.

Whole Grains

If you are used to consuming processed, fiber-poor grains like ready-to-eat cereals and white bagels on a regular basis, you may be depleting your solar plexus chakra, as you would not be getting a sustained release of energy. Additionally, refined grains seem to be trigger food for many people, since they can behave like quick-release sugars in the body. We may become easily addicted to their quick energy if not balanced by whole, unrefined grains. Whole grains like oatmeal, cooked pearled barley, bulgur, and buckwheat are superb sources of quality carbohydrates like fiber and starches. As a result, they can be an excellent food for balancing an overburdened solar plexus chakra.

Refined grains can spike blood sugar, causing one's appetite to be out of control. However, sometimes even whole grains like cooked brown rice create a similar issue. For any number of reasons, these individuals are not able to process grains efficiently. In these cases, I recommend that they refrain from grains entirely. For them, eating grains at all may unnecessarily involve the solar plexus chakra, which most likely needs strong healing and recovery. Once people get their lives into balance, they are able to better handle grains in their diet and feel less of a propensity to overdo them.

As a society, we have become used to eating grains. We may start off breakfast with pancakes, eat a sandwich for lunch, and have spaghetti for dinner. By doing so, we are inundating our solar plexus chakra with too much energy. Couple that with having to integrate all the energy coming in from the outside, and you can see that we could easily overwork our solar plexus chakra. Instead, we require the variety that other foods provide both for our physiological function and also to integrate our chakras. People who are addicted to grains tend to lead busy lives that are full of worry and stress. By bringing our lives into balance by focusing on the needs of our solar plexus chakra, we will be less prone to binging on grains.

Similar to meat from different animals, each grain has its own energetic resonance on the solar plexus chakra (see Table 6.1). In their original, unprocessed form at reasonable intake, these grains can add much to the energy of this chakra. However, when we tend to overdo them or eat them repeatedly in processed form, they can impart opposite qualities that can take away from this center.

Table 6.1   Energetic Effect of Individual Grains on the Solar Plexus

Grain	Moderate Intake Effects	Excessive Consumption Effects
Barley	Sustaining, hearty, authentic	Weighed-down, sinking feeling
Oats	Soothing, lasting, comforting	Heaviness, soggy, depressed
Rice	Balance, simplicity	Chaotic, frenetic, complex
Rye	Sharp, focused, intense	Dull, lackluster, bored, numbing
Spelt	Creative, quick, efficient	Lethargic, paralyzed
Wheat	Confident, radiating endurance	Sticky, "glue-like," bitterness, depleted

Starchy Vegetables

Starchy vegetables such as corn and potatoes are healing for the solar plexus chakra as long as their intake is not excessive; if it is, they can create imbalance. Some of the root vegetables such as turnips and beets feed the solar plexus chakra in addition to the root chakra. Others include yam, pumpkin (good for aligning sacral and solar plexus chakras), winter squash, yellow summer squash, parsnip, acorn squash, corn (cornmeal), potato (red, white, gold, sweet), taro, and yucca.

A Word about Gluten

Gluten is a protein in grains like wheat, barley, rye, spelt, and, in some cases, oats (through contamination with other grains). Some people are unable to digest gluten and, as a result, cannot eat most grains. The only grains they can eat are the ones that do not contain gluten, such as brown rice, millet, amaranth, and quinoa. On an energetic level, these folks may have difficulty integrating their lower chakras. Usually, the imbalance arises at the root chakra level, where they do not feel as though they are safe. This feeling ripples into their interactions at the solar plexus chakra. Since they do not have a foundation of safety, their power is limited and guarded. They are unable to release the strong energy of the solar plexus chakra to be effective. Likewise, the transformative energy harbored in the solar plexus chakra is not opened to the extent where it can digest gluten. These individuals tend to have other digestive imbalances as well.

In the past five to seven years, there has been an increased number of gluten-free processed products on the market. This increase could reflect a heightened number of individuals developing gluten sensitivity, or raised awareness that gluten intolerance exists at high numbers. In any case, this imbalance points us to the direction of the overall societal trends. Our root chakras are less grounded especially in light of many past and recent current world events, and our solar plexus chakra is probably more spent than ever before in the past century. With this combination, perhaps it comes as no surprise that we have become incapable of digesting gluten.

It is worthwhile to note that many processed gluten-free products tend to be higher in sugar. Generally, the products that have a particular ingredient removed, such as fat, sugar, or salt, are higher in another ingredient. People following a gluten-free regimen eating store-bought products may find themselves eating greater quantities of refined sugar, which, as we discussed, is not ideal for a solar plexus chakra that requires healing.

Yellow-Colored Foods

Yellow, tan, or golden-colored foods help to bring the solar plexus into its healthy vibrating frequency. Examples of these healing foods include corn, brown rice, yellow bell pepper, yellow summer squash. Lemon juice or fresh lemon in water is an excellent tonic for an overactive liver.

Similar to the orange foods that support the sacral chakra, yellow-colored foods provide nutritious carotenoid pigments like lutein, which allow the solar plexus chakra to radiate. The common nutritional theme underlying all foods supporting the lower chakras is antioxidants, often viewed as the nutritional defenders or protectors of the body. These are the active components in foods that support all three of the body or lower chakras (root, sacral, and solar plexus chakras). The body needs these antioxidants as a way of establishing itself as separate and distinct from the external environment. These compounds symbolically provide the protection that these centers need.

The yellow or beige color of foods also represents the presence of starch, which is broken down for energy in the body by organs associated with the solar plexus chakra.

AFFIRMATIONS TO HEAL THE SOLAR PLEXUS CHAKRA

Affirmations are helpful tools that assist us in changing core belief patterns. By writing these words or by saying them on a daily basis, we infuse our subconscious with new patterns. As we continue to make them a part of our surroundings, so will they become part of who we are. Make up your own as you see appropriate. Here are some to get you started.

- *I eat foods that open me to my powerful self.*
- *The sweetness of life fills me.*
- *My internal radiance shines forth.*
- *I am balanced.*
- *The carbohydrates I eat generate harmony within me.*

FOOD AND EATING ACTIVITIES TO BALANCE THE SOLAR PLEXUS CHAKRA

- Determine if and which foods have "power" over you. For example, do you feel drawn to eat certain foods to give you energy? Are there foods you would cave in to? Do some foods make you feel "powerless" after you eat them because they have robbed you of your vital energy? Try for yourself to explore your power relationship with foods and see if you can come up with solutions to become more power-full without the use of food.
- Examine the sweetness level in your life. Give it a score from 1 to 10 with 10 being most sweet and full of joy. What does your score say? Does your sweetness level need adjustment? List five things other than food that nourish your solar plexus chakra's need for sweetness.
- Make a list of where your energy is being spent when it comes to foods and eating. Note whether you overeat, don't eat enough, or eat rapidly. Do you spend too much time preparing meals or too little? Do you rush in and out of the grocery store, or do you find yourself in a time warp, getting lost in the multitude of aisles of products?
- Do you eat mindlessly? What do you find yourself *doing* or even *thinking* while eating? Observe what brings you into focus and concentration when eating.
- Practice mindful eating with one item of food daily.

- Experience food as poetry. Write a food and eating haiku (five syllables first verse, seven syllables second verse, five syllables last verse). Here is an example:

  Strawberry divine
  Like a living heart blossom
  Each bite full of joy

- Journal a page on how stress jeopardizes your eating. Think of three ways to combat stress, and implement one per week. How do you feel at the end of the month? What in your life has shifted?

Yellow, Tan, and Golden Foods to Nourish the Solar Plexus Chakra

Fruits	Vegetables	Legumes	Grains
Bananas	Corn	Garbanzo beans	Amaranth
Grapefruits	Ginger	Lentils	Brown rice
Lemons	Yellow bell peppers	Yellow split peas	Cornmeal
Pineapples	Yellow string beans		Millet
Plantains	Yellow summer squash		Quinoa
	Yukon gold potatoes		Whole grain breads
			Whole grain cereals

Mindful Eating Exercise

Hold in your hands a raisin. Close your eyes and feel its texture. Feel the power locked within its wrinkled structure. The goodness of the sun's rays embedded into every ridge. Now open your eyes and look at it carefully not in a mode of observation, but with a loving gaze held by eyes of understanding. See the poetry in this dynamic raisin. Think back to when it was a supple grape and now how fragile it has become. How has it traveled to you and where has it traveled from? How did it connect to the larger whole of the plant it was a part of? Feel the interconnectedness it embodies and take this in through your eyes. Now put it in your mouth and before starting to chew, feel the sensation on your tongue. Does it impart any sweetness right away? What are the messages it unlocks with every bite? What does it tell you? See how many times you can chew the single raisin, being mindful of each bite. Before swallowing, think of something you want more of in your life, like "balance" and infuse the energy of "balance" into the dissolved matrix of raisin. Swallow and imagine taking in all the nutritional and spiritual goodness of the raisin, including its origins, and use it as a bridge to connect you with all of creation.

EATING PLAN TO SUPPORT POWER AND TRANSFORMATION

Food provides a vehicle for energy. Through our ability to transform foods, we can create inner power. Be in tune with your body's ability to digest through your awareness of your solar plexus chakra. These meals will nourish your solar plexus chakra and give you the energy you need.

Breakfast Options

Steel-cut oats cooked in soymilk, topped with agave nectar
Toasted rye bread with peanut butter and sliced banana
Whole grain (high-fiber) blueberry muffin with almond butter
Brown Rice Pudding*
Mixed Muesli*

Lunch Options

Falafel in a sprouted grain pita with fresh spinach leaves and sliced
    tomato, drizzled with tahini
Mediterranean Polenta Medallions*
Sunny Corn Salad*
Cup of Fiery Curry Lentil Soup* with Quinoa-Amaranth Pine Nut
    Salad*
Fresh crisp vegetables (carrots, celery, yellow squash, bell pepper)
    and garlic hummus

---

* Indicates recipe at back of book

Dinner Options

Brown rice pasta with pine nuts, stir-fried yellow squash, bell pepper
Wild rice pilaf with light roasted garbanzo beans and corn
Curried cauliflower with cubed golden potatoes and cashews
Power Brown Rice with Yellow Vegetables and Sesame-Tahini Dressing*
and grilled chicken

CHAPTER 7

FOODS FOR LOVE
AND COMPASSION

Feeding the Heart Chakra

*It is only with the heart that one can see rightly; what is
essential is invisible to the eye.*
—ANTOINE DE SAINT-EXUPERY

Air • Depth • Unconditional Love • Gratitude • Joy •
Emotional Wisdom • Empathy • Devotion • Loyalty •
Dedication • Forgiveness • Unification

MELANIE: A LOSS OF HEART

At the age of six, Melanie lost her father to pancreatic cancer. It was a tragic, quick death that left Melanie reeling with emotions. Her mother was quite grief stricken and was not able to give Melanie the comfort or attention that she needed at the time. Instead, Melanie's mother chose to push past her hurt and to enter into a new relationship with a very abusive man. Melanie was frightened by her mother's new lover and spent much time tucked away in her small bedroom on her own. In the years that followed, Melanie became more of a loner, spending time away from home whenever possible. She found ways to keep herself busy and distracted, usually by staying late after school and by losing herself in fiction at the local library.

As an adult, Melanie found herself unable to truly connect with others, even in intimate relationships. In conversations, she felt disconnected in a way that made it difficult for her to relate to anyone. Her feelings remained stifled and stagnant. She often thought that if she began crying she wouldn't be able to stop. Therefore, it was safer for her not to feel. Melanie didn't take very good care of her body and ate poorly. She preferred to eat alone. In her forties, she developed breathing difficulties that later turned into asthma. At her core, Melanie lost sight of what it meant to feel. She was able only to tap into the loneliness and isolation she felt since her father's death.

Melanie displays the true extreme of the imbalanced heart chakra in that throughout her whole life lies a woven thread of grief and sorrow. Her emotions remained lodged somewhere in the caverns of her heart rather than being expressed. In turn, her heart has become stagnant, similar to that experienced with a blocked sacral chakra, only with a deeper and more profound effect. These trapped feelings strongly influence her ability to give and receive love. One of the ways to heal this deep grief and pain is to bring the emotion to the surface to express it as it chooses to come out. This act is typically done in a nurturing, supportive environment. In Melanie's case, her emotions were glossed over by family members close to her, so she had not learned how to express deep, heartfelt emotions.

When we allow the emotions to run free when they are felt, the energy flow can resume once again from the sacral chakra to the heart chakra. In Melanie's case, many emotions had remained "incomplete," meaning they had never finished their course or come full circle. They are like live, electrical wires that sting if they are not capped and closed. Eventually, these unfinished, unexpressed emotions end up being lodged in the fabric of our being and manifest as a disease in the physical body. For Melanie, this lack of expression resulted in asthma, or rather, in her ability to surrender to the breath of life. Her path to healing involved completing her stored emotions first by acknowledging them in the open and then honoring them in whatever form she felt called to, such as in a poem, prayer, or even physical movement.

THE HEART CHAKRA: EMOTIONS

UNHEALTHY HEART CHAKRA INDICATIONS

Melanie's situation represents one manifestation of a block in the heart chakra. See whether you have some degree of heart chakra imbalance through your responses to the following questions:

- Do you feel that you often take on people's emotions for them rather than allowing them to feel the emotions themselves?
- Do you feel your emotions to the extent that you feel trapped by them, as if they are controlling your life?
- Do you find yourself giving *others* your time or energy without giving to *yourself*?
- Do you have an aversion to eating green vegetables?
- Do you find it difficult to say "No" to others in need?
- Do you get chest pains?
- Do you have asthma or similar breathing difficulties?
- Are you fatigued from overnurturing?
- Are you resentful for overgiving? Do you feel as though you never seem to get back what you put out emotionally?
- Do you have difficulty giving and receiving love?
- Have you had a traumatic event that has left you unable to have deep feelings?
- Are you unable to express your emotions?
- Do you have difficulty with people touching you (hugging, kissing, touch on the hand or back)?
- Do you feel dispassionate about life?
- Do you feel numb?
- Do you hold back on emotions that seem to be "too much" for you?
- Are you unable to forgive yourself or others?

HEALTHY HEART CHAKRA BEHAVIOR

The heart chakra is different from the lower three chakras in that it has more of an ethereal or an air quality associated with it. When we enter heart chakra territory, it is like stepping into a realm that is on the tipping point of being more soul than body. Some traditions perceive the heart chakra as the "divining rod" between body and spirit. Indeed, the heart chakra is a much needed "Earth tool" for a spiritual being in the flesh. Healthy heart chakras use the massive love the heart pours forth as a healing salve for ourselves, others, and the planet. Therefore, it is not entirely physical, like the chakras that represent the elements of earth (root chakra), water (sacral chakra), and fire (solar plexus chakra).

When our heart chakra beats to an optimum rhythm, it will sit comfortably on a throne surrounded by love, feeling, and discernment. The heart chakra is capable of translating the raw emotions spun from the wild wheel of the sacral chakra into a tapestry of pure feeling with a basis of wisdom. We may think of someone with an "open heart" as being endlessly giving and self-sacrificing; however, a well-developed heart chakra implies loving discernment and detachment as the highest expression of love.

Similar to the solar plexus chakra, the heart chakra can easily find itself in the overdrive position of giving without the reciprocation of receiving. However, a healthy functioning heart chakra will be able to deliver feelings and love without compromising the expression of feelings and love of self. There will be clearly defined boundaries on how love is exchanged. Those who are truly heart based will put their emotions first and foremost as their guiding principle for decision making; they will, in other words, "follow their heart."

Finally, individuals with a healthy functioning heart chakra recognize the beauty and wonder of life and are patient with the process of life. They feel joy, contentment, and gratitude. No hint of stress is to be found on their faces. They are accepting and grateful for being able to share their love and radiate this energy to others. The Dalai Lama is the perfect example of a radiant heart chakra in the flesh. He wears a gentle smile and generates a warm, loving presence.

THE HEART REIGNS SUPREME

In traditional Chinese medicine, the heart is revered as the sovereign or the keeper of the spirit. The ancient Aztec practice of human sacrifice led to the offering of the human heart as the highest gift to the gods. In today's world, as in the past, the heart takes on a special meaning for many people. Several references regarding the heart and love are used in our everyday language: the heart symbol is plastered on t-shirts, bumper stickers, books, and so forth. The word *love* takes on a variety of meanings, all the way from romantic love to platonic love to familial love. *Love* has become a ubiquitous word: "I loved that movie!" "I love going on vacation." Without a doubt, the heart chakra is pervasive in our consciousness.

Some spiritual traditions would argue that the Earth plane of life is primarily about lessons of love and the heart. One could say that Jesus Christ and the Dalai Lama are two Divine beings whose energy resonates strongly with the heart chakra. If you take a moment to reflect, it may seem that every event in our lives is a call to love, whether an angry outburst, a teary good-bye, or bitter silence. At the root of every dysfunction is our unfulfilled need to be loved deeply. When we do not feel loved, we act out to get the attention we desire. Basking in love allows us to melt comfortably into our being. As Virgil stated, "Love conquers all."

The heart chakra, which sits deep into the center of the body at the level of the physical heart, takes on a mystical quality for most of us, for good reasons. There is now some research to perhaps indicate why we are such "heart-struck" beings; namely that our heart may, in fact, be the seat of our intelligence. Dr. Rollin McCraty has reported that the magnetic field of the heart is "around 5000 times stronger than that produced by the brain" and can be "measured several feet away from the body." Have you ever walked into a meeting and felt a sudden shot of anxiety running through your chest before anyone has uttered a word? Or before shaking hands with someone, you get an immediate impression of them as you enter the room where they are sitting? Our heart chakra enables us to "feel" situations without the need for any words or actions. It has its own "sixth sense." When we receive the sensory and emotional information from the heart chakra, we can take it in further and process it through our higher third eye chakra, which oversees our intuition and insight. Most people would like to think that it's the brain that gives us our sense of perception; however, emerging research is revealing that the heart's ability has been grossly underestimated.

> A well-developed heart chakra implies loving discernment and detachment as the highest expression of love.

HEALING COMES FROM THE HEART

When our heart chakra connects to our other chakras, our being takes on an even, rhythmic pattern of coherence, or the synchronization of energy. In this state, we become a wellspring of heartfelt love and joy. When we love, we create a flow of abundant healing energy running through us, connecting us with a person or a population. Studies have shown that health practitioners can be more effective when they come from a place of compassion rather than no compassion and love at all. Larry Dossey, M.D., has commented that "the majority of healing studies suggests that a healing effect is real and mediated by compassion and empathy."

Love melts resentment, anger, and bitterness and turns them into a beautiful landscape of forgiveness and joy. One of the largest blocks to love is not being able to forgive. Forgiveness is the ability to let go of the past and any regrets and acts like floodgates, allowing love to pour in. Since love is such a big deal for us human beings, it is no wonder that so many of our health issues are related to the heart. Heart disease continues to be the number one killer of both men and women. When we block our ability to forgive, we block our arteries. We get high cholesterol. We eventually get heart attacks. Through connecting with the love inside us, we soften our hearts and keep our circulation of blood moving healthily.

Core Issues Associated with the Heart Chakra

• Ability to be thankful to self, others, and God
• Ability to express love
• Expressing feelings as they arise in a constructive manner
• Loving a higher spiritual presence
• Loving others
• Loving the self
• Putting boundaries on feelings and their expression

GIVING AND RECEIVING

All of the chakras are responsible for giving out energy and for taking it in. As we discussed in chapter 6, the solar plexus chakra is a large interface for the exchange of opinions, beliefs, judgments, and ideas between the internal and external worlds. Similarly, the heart chakra is about the capacity to give and receive love.

The messages our society sends out hint at an open, giving heart as being a healthy thing, which it can be. When we hear expressions such as "openhearted," "big-hearted," "warmhearted," we may think of an individual who possesses beneficial qualities such as kindness, generosity, and being loving. However, the heart chakra is not a one-way street of love. The important piece that may often be lost in translation in such phrases is that the heart chakra has its own wisdom of how much to give and receive. As you may imagine, repeated giving without balancing with receiving can lead to "compassion fatigue." The heart chakra becomes overextended and health issues can arise.

> **When we block our ability to forgive, we block our arteries. We get high cholesterol. We eventually get heart attacks.**

The heart chakra spans a range of giving and receiving activities: compassion, empathy, dedication, loyalty, and devotion. When we empathize, we put ourselves in the other person's shoes to know what he or she may be feeling. Compassion takes place when, knowing another's feelings, we feel a surge within us to help him. Of course, we keep our heart chakra in balance by not taking on others' feelings. The heart chakra sings to the rhythm of providing a nurturing, energetic expanse in which another individual can authentically feel their emotions.

Dedication, loyalty, and devotion are the adornments of the heart. They are the jewels that allow the heart to shine its loving intention in a consistent manner.

THE NATURE OF THE LOVE VIBRATION

The heart chakra resonates primarily with the color associated with the lush nature of Mother Earth: a deep forest green or emerald. However, in some individuals, it can vibrate to the color associated with rose or pink. Sometimes, both colors are found here, with the rose color in the core, surrounded by green. Readings of the heart chakra reveal scenes of the vastness of nature, especially in those individuals with an open heart chakra. It may also be perceived as a large vortex with much depth. Divine figures of compassion, such as Christ or Kuan Yin, the Buddhist goddess of compassion, are often found within the depths of the heart chakra, along with flowers that feature a complex array of petals, such as the lotus flower or the rose. People and animal figures in our lives can be stored within the onion layers of the heart.

> **The heart chakra sings to the rhythm of providing a nurturing, energetic expanse in which another individual can authentically feel their emotions.**

PHYSIOLOGY AND THE HEART CHAKRA

As the name suggests, the heart chakra is associated primarily with the heart and lungs. The heart and lungs share an intimate relationship, as they work together for the single goal of pumping oxygen via the blood to the rest of the body. Peripheral to the heart and lungs, the heart chakra governs the breasts, shoulders, armpits, arms, wrists, and hands. The arms are essentially an extension of the heart chakra, as they are the tools needed for touch and reaching out to others. Touching is an important healing activity of the heart chakra.

Anatomy Associated with the Heart Chakra

- Armpits
- Arms
- Blood vessels
- Breasts
- Hands
- Heart
- Lungs
- Lymphatic system
- Shoulders
- Wrists

The blood vessel network throughout the body is connected to the heart chakra, as it is the means by which the blood and life force are delivered throughout the body. As we learned in chapter on the sacral chakra, the heart (fourth) chakra refines the emotions created by the sacral chakra by incorporating divine wisdom. If there is a blockage in the sacral chakra, the heart chakra will need to compensate or assist with the healing of the sacral chakra.

THE RELATIONSHIP OF LOVE AND COMPASSION TO FOODS AND EATING

With the lower chakras, food and eating are used to serve the many aspects of the body, including survival, the body's need for pleasure, and its need for transformation and energy. In the realm of the upper chakras, food and eating take on less of a physical emphasis and more of a symbolic significance. In several cultures, food is used as a vehicle to show love. Think of Valentine's Day and all the boxes of chocolates that lovers exchange. Dating couples may connect by going out to have a meal at a restaurant. Mothers bake cookies for their children. Essentially, the message we are delivering is that if we care about someone, we feel the need to share food with them, whether preparing it for them, serving it, or eating along with them. We extend the love we have through the conduit of food.

Also, it is through the act of eating that we show that we value and love the bodies we have. If we didn't care for ourselves, we would stop eating altogether (unless the act of starvation was linked to a cause). Traditions have used the adage, "Your body is your temple." Indeed, loving ourselves implies providing ourselves with constant, quality nourishment.

Most important, even though the heart chakra may not have a strong resonance with the *physical* matter of food, it comprises our inner fulcrum, from which our eating experience balances. What this means is that without a basis of love and a blossoming, beautiful, free heart chakra, we are unable to lovingly assimilate any quantity or quality of nutrients we take in, no matter how pure and adequate they may be for our physical flesh. Individuals who fixate on obtaining the proper ratio of nutrients become stuck within the realm of the lower chakras. This is not the point of nourishment: love is what liberates us and energizes every particulate we pass through our lips. When we enter into the eating experience with an open, loving heart chakra, we magnify the healing effects of foods manifold compared to eating from a place of nonlove. The greatest nourishment we can ever take in is that of love. Love infuses every morsel of food we ingest. Without it, we starve our hearts, and ultimately, our soul.

> The greatest nourishment we can ever take in is that of love. Love infuses every morsel of food we ingest. Without it, we starve our hearts, and ultimately, our soul.

HEART CHAKRA FOOD AND EATING HEALING PLAN

Connect to Who and What We Love Through Eating

You may have heard the phrases, "You are who you love" and "You are what you eat." When we love someone, we develop a heartfelt connection with them, like an invisible cord of energy that runs between us and them. The level of bonding can be so deep that the feelings felt by each one of us may be shared by the other, either knowingly or not. In turn, our feelings can direct how we eat. As a result, we may end up eating similarly to those we love.

This concept was demonstrated in a large published study in the *New England Journal of Medicine*. The authors, Drs. Christakis and Fowler, demonstrated that patterns of body weight gain were directly connected to our social networks. In other words, the greater the connection an individual would have with obese friends and family, even if miles apart, the larger the influence on her developing obesity. So, if your close (not necessarily physically, but emotionally close) friend was obese, there was a higher chance of you becoming obese.

In a similar way, studies have shown that children model the eating habits of their parents, particularly girls patterning their mothers. Thus, one of the best things a parent can do for his or her child is to ensure that the parent is setting a consistent example of healthy eating.

Eat and Serve Food with Love and Gratitude

Have you ever had a meal made with love, or had all of the parts of the meal carefully, lovingly created, prepared, and served to you? If you have, you will know what a treat it is and how it feeds the body along with the spirit. Love is the highest vibration possible. When food is in the presence of love, it takes on that high vibration. Infusing love into food can cause it to taste sweeter, more flavorful.

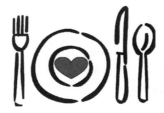

People who buy organic food claim that it tastes better than conventionally grown food when compared side by side, even when they do not know which one is which. Does organic food taste better because of the absence of pesticides and other chemicals? Probably. Does the fact that it is carefully tended to and grown in harmony with nature add to the improved flavor? Most likely. There certainly is an element of love that appears to go into organic gardening. And when we make the selection for organic food, we are actively tapping into the love that has grown into the food imparted from the sun, stars, moon, sky, farmer, harvester, and grocer.

If you haven't experienced it, or even if you have, try to feel love in every cell of your being while you are preparing food. Start by feeling love and compassion coming from the magnificent lotus of your heart chakra with every slice, simmer, and sauté, to see whether you notice the difference throughout your body and in your energy level. Chances are that if you are preparing food with love and eating it with love, you will feel a warm kindness radiate through you while eating and after eating, due to the opening of the heart chakra responding to the love in the food. The food particles are receptive to this energy and will absorb it immediately.

Similarly, how do we respond to a meal that is prepared with love? How do we express gratitude for food? There is a high level of ritual that corresponds with eating. Some religions and spiritual practices include a prayer, grace, or offering of gratitude at the beginning of a meal. It may begin at the hunt for an animal, giving thanks to the animal for sharing its life and energy with the tribe, or even at the point of picking fruits and vegetables for a meal.

Author Don Gerrard has published a book on the concept of eating from "one bowl." When we concentrate our love and intention into our eating vessel, food and eating take on an elevated meaning. We become more aware of what we are putting into our bowl and how that nurtures us. I also like people to choose a special utensil to use when eating. Sometimes I choose to eat with a small teaspoon with a rose on the handle. Doing so helps me to take in and savor small bites and the rose is a reminder of the beauty and love of foods.

Share Meals with Others

When we share love, we receive more back: the love in our hearts grows exponentially. We never go into energetic bankruptcy by sharing love. In fact, quite the opposite! In much the same way, sharing meals with others feeds our heart chakra. Cathy describes that she dreaded eating because she ate alone. Eating was not a heartfelt activity. It made her feel lonely. When I recommended that she invite others over to eat every Sunday afternoon, eating took on a whole new meaning and feeling. She looked forward to every Sunday and inviting new guests over and trying new recipes. The process of invitation to others opened her heart chakra. Food became a passion for her. She was invited as a guest to other homes and welcomed to eat in her friends' presence.

Eating in a communal setting is so important for us as human beings. We are social by nature. Our lives in a spiritual sense are about giving and receiving love. When we build walls around us, we close off the heart chakra. Eating with others can create so much joy, especially when the meals are prepared together.

Eating with others, just like praying with others, intensifies the energy received from the experience.

FOODS FOR LOVE AND COMPASSION

The lower three chakras revolve around the macronutrient universe of protein, fats, and carbohydrates. In fact, most nutrition texts hone in on these "big guns" of the dietary arena. We eat several grams of each of them every day; the sheer quantity of macronutrients makes up the bulk of our eating. However, there are some nutrients that never get to take the center stage, yet they can be as important. These nutrients are called "phytochemicals" (*phyto* means "plant"): the tiny pigments and compounds imparting color and protection to plants and health benefits to people. There are several thousands of them in our food supply, and their effects, even though their absolute quantity may be less, have significant potential.

As we journey up the chakras, the nourishment that feeds these energy centers becomes less bulky and more fine and delicate. Rather than whole, large foods, the healing properties for chakras may be the individual constituents of foods that may be invisible to the naked eye. Thus, with the increasing complexity of our energy centers—similar to an expedition into our spiritual fabric—we start to mine deeper into the matrix of our food supply.

Foods for love and compassion resonate with the diamond shape. Note the four directions, symbolizing the heart chakra as the fourth chakra. The diamond is a symbol of expansion, of growth and opening in all directions. All directions are pointing outward, like the feeling generated by love. The diamond symbolizes a leaf of a tree, green and open to the rays of the sun and the molecules of carbon dioxide, capturing the connection between plants and the heart chakra. Reflect on the amazing intricacy of plant foods that feed the heart chakra: layers of leaves bundled together in a sphere of cabbage or tiny buds full of life force clustered together into a broccoli floret. Indeed, plants are some of the most tenacious life-forms on the planet—they are confined to one place and are able to survive, a quality very similar to that of the heart chakra ("Love conquers all").

Overall, with its strong connection to nature and plants, the heart chakra resonates with vegetables and their respective "phyto" compounds: phytochemicals, phytoestrogens, phytosterols.

Vegetables

Before diving into the "phyto" territory, it is worthwhile to start with the physically large, visible food influences on the heart chakra. Essentially, vegetables, on the whole, speak clearly to the heart chakra and provide what it needs to be grounded in healthy boundaries and yet expansive and loving. However, there are select vegetables that have a deeper bond to the heart chakra.

CRUCIFEROUS VEGETABLES

Cruciferous vegetables, such as broccoli, cauliflower, and Brussels sprouts, are especially balancing for the heart chakra. The very organization of these vegetables mirrors that of the unfolding spirals of the roselike heart chakra. These vegetables are composed of several components or layers, such as broccoli, which is a crowd of tiny florets, like a forest on a stick. Brussels sprouts and onions share a similar quality, but in a different way: they are multidimensional, built up of many layers coming together.

Cruciferous Vegetables to Nourish the Heart Chakra

- Arugula
- Bok choy
- Broccoflower
- Broccoli
- Brussels sprouts
- Cabbage, Chinese
- Cabbage, green
- Cabbage, Napa
- Cabbage, red
- Cauliflower
- Collard greens
- Daikon
- Horseradish
- Kale
- Mustard greens
- Wasabi
- Watercress

The cruciferous vegetables share a common stinky, sulfur smell, indicating that they are effective at guarding the body from toxins. Sulfur-containing compounds such as sulforaphanes found in broccoli act as detoxification agents in the body. They work together with the intestines and liver (overseen by the solar plexus and sacral chakras) to rid the body of contaminants. Observe your reactions to green vegetables, as it could provide a small mirror of what is happening within your heart chakra. I have worked with several people who have damage in their heart chakra energy who will simply not eat green vegetables. Jessica states, "My parents would steam broccoli, and the smell was so awful! It would fill the house, making me feel sick." Others have commented the opposite. Simon reports, "One of the reasons I enjoy green vegetables is because I feel closer to the earth; I like their earthy flavor." It is very common to hear how good and vibrant people feel when they eat green vegetables.

Some of these greens, such as collard greens and mustard greens, are bitter and slightly astringent in taste. The bitter taste dampens excessive energy in the heart chakra, swinging it back into balance.

LEAFY GREENS

From an energy perspective, fresh leafy greens, a composite of many layers and depth, allow the heart chakra to open when eating them. These leaves are full of circulating life. The tiny weblike imprint embedded into their matrix resembles the circulatory system that the heart chakra oversees as part of her kingdom. They literally feed us with life force, aliveness, and freshness.

On a physical level, fresh leafy salad greens contain nutrients like folate and vitamin K to keep our heart chakra protected and aligned with other chakras. Folate is important for the reproduction and maintenance of cells. It is needed for DNA replication, suggesting that it is a key nutrient for bridging together the cellular life force from our ancestry that's woven into the DNA from the root chakra with the destiny we create for ourselves, depending on the lives we lead through our heart chakra. Also, folate is one of the protectors against high levels of a compound called *homocysteine,* which is associated with injury to the blood vessels.

Vitamin K, another building block of greens, creates an energy linkage from the heart chakra to the root chakra through its role in bone metabolism. Its other job is to oversee the flow of blood. Without adequate vitamin K, we would not be able to clot blood appropriately to prevent us from bleeding in case of an injury or accident. Vitamin K, from the lens of the energy world, keeps the heart chakra safe within the confines of our energetic being. This is a noteworthy function, especially since the nature of the heart chakra is to expand and release. Without a protective mechanism in place, we would bleed energetically if we did not have essential nutrients like vitamin K in our food.

Finally, leafy salad greens like romaine, red leaf, butterhead (Bibb), escarole, iceberg, and spinach are perfect to eat during the lunch time, when the sun is at its peak, which also coincides with the time that our internal "metabolic fire" burns brightest. These greens keep us calm, cool, and collected in the midst of external and internal "fire" that can be very damaging to the tender heart chakra.

SPROUTS

In much the same way as the leafy greens, sprouts impart a young life-force energy of renewal to the heart chakra. Eating them helps us to better connect with the "inner child"—the playful, innocent, pure part of us that lives within our heart chakra. Young sprouts, whether broccoli, alfalfa, or mung, to name a few, are truly the dancing molecules of energy our heart cherishes. Because of the abundance of live, active enzymes they contain, sprouts can assist us in more colorfully assimilating life, releasing us from any heavy burden we may feel in this area.

RAW FOODS

The cooling properties of raw foods allow the heart chakra to come into balance if it is fueled with too much fiery energy. In some individuals, the heart chakra is vulnerable to the "heat" of unexpressed, raw emotions from the sacral chakra. When we open ourselves to expressing emotions, our heart chakra rides a wave of calm. If not, we set our heart aflame. For emotional upheavals, adopting a raw food regimen may be helpful to allow your energetic body to release and process lodged thoughts and feelings.

Fresh salads full of leafy greens and sprouts are an excellent base upon which to build your base of raw foods. Even aiming for one raw foods meal daily could alleviate emotional avalanches over the long term!

Phytochemicals

Researchers have slowly been uncovering the population of phytochemicals within our foods. M. C. Walsh and colleagues estimate that there are up to 10,000 of these found in the layers of fruits, vegetables, whole grains, and legumes. Just think of the potential effect of these thousands of compounds individually and in concert on our physiology and our energetic self! And to think that we may limit ourselves to the silos of the three nutritional musketeers: protein, fat, and carbohydrate.

Many times, these phytochemicals are what give plants their color. For example, lycopene is the phytochemical that makes a tomato red; beta-carotene is what makes carrots orange. These and other potent phytochemicals are what is missing from the "brown, yellow, and white" foods of the Standard American Diet.

Moreover, phytochemicals are not just about looking pretty by adding color. They serve particular physiological functions within the body. Our bodies are not enlightened enough to create all the nutrients we need. These phytochemical helpers keep our physiology and spiritual beings strung together and glowing with life. The heart chakra starves without these phytochemicals, and when our heart is ravaged, our whole soul self is depleted and empty. Look at the age of industrialization that we entered into in the past hundred years. Our food supply has been stripped of color-full, purpose-full, Divinely crafted plant compounds and replaced with human-made ratios and proportions of synthetic nutrients ("fortification"). Clearly, this is a regression from our higher chakras into our lower chakras, as there is an intellectualization on the part of humans who think that they know what is best rather than trusting the wisdom of nature, of the Divine.

With our outpouring of phytochemically depleted foods and lackluster energy (think of our current society as a hyperactive solar plexus chakra spewing forth copious external energy), we have become, quite sadly, empty of heart. We regain our heart chakra strength by eating foods of color and complexity. Foods that are grown organically produce different phytochemicals to make them hearty in a stressful environment. Eating plant foods, particularly those of the rainbowed, organic, unprocessed variety, brings our heart back into happy mode. When our heart chakra resonates with our highest frequency, we can better take in and assimilate other foods.

CHLOROPHYLL

An example of an incredibly power-full, heart-loving phytochemical is that of chlorophyll, which could perhaps be coined "king of the phytochemicals." High-chlorophyll foods such as spirulina, wheat grass, and chlorella are nourishing for the heart chakra through their positive health effects on the blood and circulation. Chlorophyll is the building block of all plants and is responsible for transforming light into energy for the plant cell. Similarly, it brings universal light to our cells, while at the same time protecting the cells from ultraviolet (UV) ray damage by acting as an antioxidant protector.

Whereas the solar plexus chakra is responsible for bringing in and putting out energy, the heart chakra oversees the entire being. Symbolically, it is the sovereign sitting in its throne, guiding and protecting its cellular and spirit kingdom. In much the same way, high-chlorophyll foods provide us with our ancestral essence, including all the building blocks required on a primordial level. Ingestion of high-chlorophyll foods is one way to bridge the gap between the purely physical and primal survival nature of the root chakra and the spirit connection that resides in the heart.

The heart chakra kingdom needs troops to stand on guard to defend against invaders. Chlorophyll provides the necessary nutritional guard to bind toxins so that they can be excreted. As a result, the blood remains pure and free of contaminants, and the overall system is protected. Additionally, foods high in chlorophyll are cooling and anti-inflammatory, probably due to their antioxidant action. Overall, all green-colored foods will contain chlorophyll and can be ingested for their ability to keep out invading microorganisms.

Foods Rich in Chlorophyll

- Alfalfa grass
- Barley grass
- Chlorella
- Green vegetables
- Spirulina
- Wheatgrass

PHYTOESTROGENS

Since the heart chakra holds within her kingdom the breast region, it is worth considering eating plant foods that contain compounds that support breast health and hormone balance, depending on your health condition. There are certain foods, such as soybeans, red clover, and flaxseed, which are rich in plant compounds that resemble the hormone estrogen. These compounds are referred to as *phytoestrogens,* or plant estrogens. Even though they look like estrogen and can bind to the same receptors on a cell as estrogen, they are not as potent as estrogen. They have only a fraction of estrogen's activity. Their consumption has been shown to be linked to protection against prostate, breast, and other cancers, cardiovascular disease, and possibly even osteoporosis and menopausal symptoms.

Our bodies try to put us into balance and give us the right amount of hormones, but sometimes we may end up with too little or too much. When we eat one of the several types of plant foods that contain phytoestrogens, we may be able to change our hormone levels and their action in the body. The receptors for estrogen located on cells throughout the body, including the breast and reproductive (sacral chakra territory for women, root chakra turf in men) tissue, are sensitive to the presence of dietary estrogens. Since dietary phytoestrogens mimic estrogen's activity to some degree, they can act as a substitute and bind weakly to estrogen receptors on estrogen-sensitive tissues. As a result, they prevent the more potent estrogen compound from binding to the tissue. This action can be beneficial when we have too much estrogen in the body. On the other hand, when we have very little estrogen in the body, eating soy and flax products may provide an estrogenic effect in the body.

In healthy individuals, plant foods containing phytoestrogens may help keep breast tissue, or the heart chakra, vibrant. However, as you can imagine, there is debate and inconclusive evidence as to whether foods high in phytoestrogens should be consumed by individuals who have or have had cancer that is estrogen-responsive.

PHYTOSTEROLS

Phytosterols ("plant sterols") are a particular type of heart-loving phytochemical that looks similar to cholesterol but doesn't have the bad rap of cholesterol. In fact, there is much information stacking in favor of the health-promoting characteristics of these constitutive plant compounds. Phytosterols are naturally found in virtually all plant foods, including nuts, seeds, whole grains, and vegetables. Their primary role is to block cholesterol absorption in the body and to keep cell membranes healthy.

Because they are found in a variety of different plant foods that resonate with other chakras, phytosterols are an excellent example of how the chakras can be integrated through foods. One example of a plant food that contains an array of heart chakra-healing properties is the mighty avocado. In particular, it nourishes the heart and sacral chakras through its healing yellow-green color imparted by phytochemical pigments like lutein and chlorophyll (heart chakra), protective phytosterols (heart chakra), and also high levels of monounsaturated fats, which would speak to both the sacral chakra (oils) and to the heart chakra (heart-protective quality of these oils).

> A plant food that contains an array of heart chakra-healing properties is the mighty avocado.

Green-Colored Foods

As we have already discussed, the heart chakra vibrates to the frequency of green-colored foods, so the presence of or ingestion of these foods will allow the heart chakra to express to its fullest. A lush green color vibrates with the frequency of life on Earth, and therefore, it can bring the heart chakra back to its mission to cultivate love as healing throughout the Earth kingdom.

AFFIRMATIONS TO HEAL THE HEART CHAKRA

Affirmations are helpful tools that assist us in changing core belief patterns. By writing these words or by saying them on a daily basis, we infuse our subconscious with new patterns. As we continue to make them a part of our surroundings, so will they become part of who we are. Make up your own as you see appropriate. Here are some to get you started.

- *I feed my heart with dark, green leafy vegetables.*
- *I serve myself with love and acceptance.*
- *I infuse love and gratitude into the food I eat and serve to others.*
- *I give thanks to the plants and animals who gave their lives up for me.*
- *The child in me lives through eating live foods.*

Green Foods to Nourish the Heart Chakra

Vegetables		Fruits	Legumes
Artichoke	Dandelion greens	Avocado	Green beans
Arugula	Green onions	Grapes, green	Great Northern beans
Asparagus	Green peas	Honeydew melon	Green split peas
Bitter melon	Green pepper	Kiwi	Soybeans (edamame)
Bok choy	Kale	Pear	
Broccoflower	Leafy greens		
Broccoli	Leek		
Brussels sprouts	Mixed greens		
Cabbage, Chinese	Mustard greens		
Cabbage, green	Olives, green		
Cabbage, savoy	Romaine		
Celery	Snap peas		
Chard, rainbow	Spinach		
Chard, red	Sprouts (of all types)		
Collard greens	Watercress		
Cucumber	Zucchini		

FOOD AND EATING ACTIVITIES TO
BALANCE THE HEART CHAKRA

- Have a serving of green vegetables, either 1 cup of fresh salad greens, or $^1/_2$ cup of steamed broccoli or Brussels sprouts, at least once daily. Note whether you have any resistance or whether you welcome this action. How do you *feel* when you eat these greens?
- Create a prayer of gratitude and grace to say before your meals.
- Sing while you prepare food. Sound is the vehicle for the heart chakra to open. By opening your heart before eating, you may notice a greater love exchange between you and the food.
- Focus on your breath while eating, and synchronize your breath to your rhythm of eating. Breathe deeply and chew thoroughly. What messages of the heart of the food are you unlocking with every bite?
- Make a meal with love and share with a person you love. How does it taste? Does it taste differently than a meal not made with love?
- Put heart stickers all over your food packaging and containers (for example, water bottle) to remind yourself to love yourself and your food. The association of the heart symbol with its meaning of love will lead to transformation of the food.
- Eat one raw food meal daily for one week. Note whether you feel differently by the end of the week.
- Do you use food to show love? Have others used food to show love to you? How has this been beneficial or detrimental? What are alternate ways to show love?

EATING PLAN TO SUPPORT LOVE

Choose meals from each of these categories in order to complete your heart chakra needs.

Breakfast Options

Warm flaxseed meal cereal with soy milk
Soy yogurt and a shot of wheatgrass
Love-infused green grapes with sesame seed mochi
Flax-Zucchini Muffin of Joy*

---

* Indicates recipe at back of book

Lunch Options

The Heart Salad*

Cruciferous vegetables and fresh guacamole

Sesame Kale and Spinach Tango*

Thank You Rice Paper Rolls*

Dinner Options

Green Garbanzo Beans with Love Rice*

Heart-y Split Pea Soup* with spinach tortilla

Pesto pasta with broccoli florets

Heart-Warming Brussels Sprouts*

Rosemary Roasted Cauliflower and Pine Nuts*

CHAPTER 8

FOODS FOR COMMUNICATION AND TRUTH

Feeding the Throat Chakra

One's philosophy is not best expressed in words;
it is expressed in the choices one makes.
—ELEANOR ROOSEVELT

Truth • Speaking • Self-Knowledge • Hearing • Smell •
Taste • Sound • Choice • Authenticity • Communication •
Surrender • Verbal Expression • Faith

BILL: NOTHING BUT NOISE

Recently, Bill was asked by his manager to conduct computer training classes with large audiences. Upon hearing this news, Bill felt an uneasy tickling feeling in his throat, as there is a part of him that does not feel comfortable speaking in front of others. He does not want to fail but knows that he also does not want to turn down the opportunity to please his boss. Throughout his life, he has struggled with these and other choices, small and large. He has not been able to locate his "inner voice." Often, he looks outside of himself for validation and for help making decisions. Periodically, he reflects back on past decisions that he regrets and has difficulty forgetting and moving on from. His indecisiveness haunts him occasionally.

One of the reservations Bill has about public speaking is that he realizes that he has some degree of speech difficulty. He notes that he frequently mixes words together inadvertently. Also, when he was a child, his mother had him take speech therapy; Bill felt ashamed for being unable to communicate effectively. To the observer, Bill speaks rapidly, and sometimes he mumbles and rambles on in the presence of others simply to fill the space.

Similarly, he eats to fill his time, even when he is not hungry. He feels uncomfortable with silence when with others, and also when he is alone. If at home by himself, he will surround himself with the sounds of the television and radio. He quickly gulps his food, not paying attention to what he is eating. He has a lingering memory of almost choking to death when he was four years old.

Bill has a number of issues that center on the throat chakra. The most obvious ones are those related to his ability to communicate. Speaking has not always been fluid for him. Bill's throat chakra is in overdrive with his fast talking and mixing-up of words. A part of him is unwilling to take in sensory input; instead, he blocks it by talking excessively. There is an imbalance between sharing words and listening. Individuals like Bill may be thought of as those who like to "listen to themselves talk," but what is actually happening is they are preventing any valuable insightful information from entering their energetic space. On a deeper level, there may be things they do not want to hear. When we refuse to take in and acknowledge information, whether from others or from Divine guidance, we are not open to the flow of life and our highest good. Our speech reflects whether we are in sync with this flow or not.

People like Bill pad their lives with sound, creating an artificial bubble of safety and control around their lives. For Bill, the lack of clarity in his speech has cascaded into his lack of decisiveness in making choices. He is not aligned with his authentic truth and passion and with what feeds him. He is concerned with pleasing his boss only. Because of this misalignment, he dissipates his energy—a simple reflection of this loss is seen by his garbled words and mumbling. True healing for Bill will occur when he is ready to choose to be authentic and to align his will with that of the Divine.

THE THROAT CHAKRA: COMMUNICATION

UNHEALTHY THROAT CHAKRA INDICATIONS

If you answer "Yes" to the following questions, you may have a throat chakra imbalance:

* Do you express your thoughts, emotions, and feelings in a very forceful manner?
* Are you extremely talkative, to the degree that some people might say you are rambling, without making sense?
* Do you find it difficult to listen to others because you are busy expressing your own thoughts and ideas?
* Do you get very upset when life doesn't seem to be going your way?
* Do you tend to overeat when you are not hungry?
* Do you gulp your food?
* Do you feel that you have a high metabolism?
* Do you have or have you had bulimia?
* Is your voice extremely high or low pitched?
* Do you have a tendency to stutter or to mix up your words?
* Do you have difficulty expressing your thoughts, feelings, ideas, needs, or emotions?
* When attempting to express yourself, does your voice become raspy, or does it become "all choked up"?
* Do you find it overwhelmingly difficult to speak your truth for fear of punishment?
* Do you have a slow metabolism?
* Do you feel completely out of control regarding the decisions that you need to make in your life?
* Have you had or do you have anorexia or feel resistance to eating?

HEALTHY THROAT CHAKRA BEHAVIOR

A healthy functioning throat chakra will serve as the portal to communicate and express the emotions, thoughts, and feelings of the other chakras through sound in a way that is authentic and true. Communication through the throat chakra unfolds in a delicate yet firm, honest manner. There is no room for lies or deceit. When we are in alignment with our throat chakra, our words will be congruent with our actions. When we say "Yes," we mean *yes* from a place of truth. Likewise, when we speak true from our heart, we will be able to discern whether others are telling the truth. We will develop the ability to "read between the lines" of what others are trying to say.

Throat chakras that are open and flowing in harmony with the rest of the energy field will be able to provide us with discernment in *how* we express ourselves. We will have the internal knowingness to speak our truth from a place of wisdom and grace rather than from a place of blame, hurt, or resentment. We will not be prone to use cutting words to slice someone's self-esteem. Instead, we will have the wisdom to use language in a way that will empower the other. Right use of language fits with a healthy throat chakra. For example, if someone is being wrongfully accused of certain actions, the throat chakra will enable the voice to speak the truth of the situation in the way that is best for all involved, in order to remedy the condition.

A high-vibrating throat chakra will have all of its senses open and ready to experience the world it lives in. It will be able and eager to communicate these sensations received into higher learning for the self. Finally, a throat chakra that is operating on the highest level will be congruent with the needs of the Divine and will be able to release all fear, doubt, and control regarding decisions to be made in our lives. If life takes an unexpected turn, individuals with healthy throat chakras will be able to embrace this new path with acceptance, knowing that it was crafted for their highest experience.

GATEWAY TO HIGHER COMMUNICATION

Like the name suggests, the throat chakra dwells deep in our throat. This center is dense with an array of many essential body functions, such as talking, hearing, chewing, swallowing, and breathing. The messenger of the throat chakra, the voice, allows us to express our original spirit and ego formed by our solar plexus chakra and the love and wisdom of our heart chakra. As we travel up the chakra tree, each chakra becomes more complex and combines elements of the lower chakras into its highest expressions. The throat chakra does that with all of the chakras below it and has an intimate relationship with the root and solar plexus chakras. The will to survive nestled in the root chakra is complemented with the manifestation of our survival in the physical world through the solar plexus chakra.

The throat chakra goes one step beyond into the realm of higher choices and higher will. It incorporates and reminds us of the role of a Higher Presence in our lives and in the paths we choose. The throat chakra begs us to release control and to dive head on into whatever we are presented with utmost confidence that it is the best possible situation for us.

Where the heart chakra equips us with love and touch for healing, the throat chakra enables us with the senses of hearing, smelling, and tasting. It gives us the tools we need to experience and enjoy the Earth playground. Through our senses, our experience is made real, and we can learn and go on to make more choices to direct our path.

Also, the throat chakra is a center where we can be vulnerably powerful. It gives us the equipment to choose in every moment. When we are not aware of this tremendous choice, we lose our power and remain unaware and unawake. We make ourselves known through the throat chakra, by maximizing the connection of the physical body to the ethereal spirit. The actions of the throat chakra may be linked to our highest potential and good. It is a key chakra for minorities, and individuals and groups whose rights have been suppressed on an individual basis or on the whole. With the voice it provides, we can choose to liberate ourselves from the bonds of others. In essence, the throat chakra continually presents us with a crossroads at which we get to select our path.

If an individual harbors within her physical or spiritual fabric residual memories of being restricted or prohibited from speaking her voice and making her own choices, these blocks will reveal themselves in the throat chakra. The neck is a delicate part of the body—a portal for spirit to enter the physical body. Throughout time, there have been a number of ways to sever the neck, whether through hanging or using a guillotine. Symbolically, the human approach to attempting to control various situations has involved this means of destroying the entry of spirit.

Mary states that she feels the need to keep her neck secure by wearing scarves or turtlenecks. If someone confronts her, she senses a tingling constriction around her neck. Past-life regression work revealed that she was killed for her expressing her belief systems by severing her throat. Thus, the energy that we carry with us can definitely influence our present-day chakras.

AUTHENTICITY

At your core, who are you and what do you stand for? What does your true self look like, not just as a body but also as a spiritual being? The throat chakra welcomes us to use the courage of the heart to put a stake in the ground of our beliefs, opinions, feelings, and thoughts. It gives us the tool of will to move in the direction of our authenticity. When we do not act authentically, it is like throwing away the gifts of the throat chakra.

SURRENDER

The solar plexus chakra endows us with our personal will to make choices, and the throat chakra is responsible for integration of our personal will with Divine will. This means that when we are about to choose or move forward in a direction, the throat chakra helps to step back from the situation to see how this act connects with what is intended for us by Spirit. Our aim is to ultimately be in alignment with our highest purpose and good, which is Divine will.

Stepping back and surrendering to a decision is easy to say, but it may be trying for most people. Since many individuals have solar plexus chakra issues, it's no doubt that our natures have gravitated toward being more controlling. It is challenging to allow someone or some force to step in and tell you how your life needs to be lived. And that's where surrender comes in. Surrender allows us to fall backward into the arms of God. The throat chakra helps us to let go of all attachment to outcome and live our life as it mystically unfolds before us.

Core Issues Associated with the Throat Chakra

- Accepting the path provided to us by a higher spiritual presence
- Acknowledgment of a higher spiritual presence
- Being able to verbally express needs, emotions, thoughts, and feelings in a way that serves the self
- Releasing control and accepting life
- Speaking one's personal truth
- Utilizing the senses for obtaining learning from their experience

---

THE NATURE OF THE COMMUNICATION VIBRATION

Compared with the heart chakra, which is abundant with earthly fixtures, the throat chakra allows for a turning away from the Earth self and a tilting toward the blue sky, away from all that is limiting and directed inward. The throat chakra resonates with the color of sky, a pale to deep aquamarine. Readings of this center are sometimes associated with flying images such as winged creatures or objects. It allows for more fantasy-type objects, such as flying dragons, than do some of the lower chakras. Depending on the health of the throat chakra, either images of freedom and flying or constriction and suffocation may come through.

PHYSIOLOGY OF THE THROAT CHAKRA

As the name suggests, the throat chakra works with the throat and the anatomy surrounding the throat, including the larynx, pharynx, thyroid, neck, upper esophagus, chin, tongue, lips, mouth, ears, and nose. The ability of the nose to smell, the tongue to taste, and the ears to hear are all contained within the throat chakra vicinity. The throat chakra is essential for our connection to food. To a large degree, we experience food through our throat chakra by smelling and tasting it, chewing it, and coating it with saliva, which assists in the breakdown of certain nutrients, and finally, swallowing it and making it accessible to the rest of the body. Our intent for that food is set within the throat chakra, and the throat chakra determines and chooses foods that are needed for our highest good.

Anatomy Associated with the Throat Chakra

• Cheeks	• Mouth	• Throat
• Chin	• Neck	• Tongue
• Ears	• Nose	• Upper esophagus
• Larynx	• Pharynx	
• Lips	• Thyroid gland	

The throat chakra also governs to a great extent how we will process our food, since it contains within it the thyroid, the gland responsible for our basal metabolism. Separate from our interaction with food, the throat chakra provides us with the anatomical machinery to utter a sound and to create words using the air we breathe through our mouth and nose. Finally, another core function of the throat chakra is to enable us to breathe, and by doing so, we accept life and surrender to it.

THE RELATIONSHIP OF COMMUNICATION
AND TRUTH TO FOODS AND EATING

The higher chakras (from the heart chakra upward) are more about our *relationship* with foods and eating rather than about the foods themselves. The throat chakra is very much about authentic connection with food; it equips us with the processes we need, such as chewing, tasting, hearing, and speaking, to enrich our relationship with food and eating. It is a dense area with much activity happening all at once. Therefore, it is important for us to work with this chakra to make the highest choices at all times, especially those involving foods and eating.

OUR SENSORY RELATIONSHIP WITH FOODS

As we discussed in chapter 5, on the sacral chakra, humans are sensory beings. We take in sensory information and process it on many levels. For the sacral chakra, we use the sensory input for pleasure. For the solar plexus chakra, we receive messages from our environment that we integrate within our own energy and body. The heart chakra takes in a huge amount of emotional information in a large span of space even before any interaction has taken place. The throat chakra represents a practical manifestation of our sensory tools.

The narrow space governed by the throat chakra is dense with our body sensors: our ears, nose, lips, tongue, and mouth. We are able to use these sensors to a significant degree with foods and eating. In fact, all of these sensors are engaged when we eat.

Our ears give us the capacity to listen intently to communication about eating, whether listening for animals when hunting in the wild or to the screeching of the tea kettle boiling water on the stove. Eating is about receiving, and the throat chakra helps us to do that with our ears. What do we hear as we shop at the grocery store? Some of us have our little throat chakra antics that we enjoy in food selection: shaking melons, pounding gently on an acorn squash. In the more subtle background, our sensory experience of eating may be colored by hearing "old tapes" of expectations and "I should" statements playing in the theater of our conscious mind when we shop for groceries or are selecting a food choice in a restaurant—"I really *should* have the salmon and not the rib-eye steak," "My mom would want me to eat *right*," "What would Jack say if he knew I indulged in Rocky Road ice cream?"

Sometimes, we can almost hear the person's voice resonating their message in our ears. The throat chakra encourages us to listen to our own voice when it comes to food and eating—what is real for us—rather than taking on outdated messages from others.

What about the communication exchanged in the course of eating a meal that indicates we are enjoying eating? At our best, we resort to making less noticeable sounds while eating to convey our enjoyment. Think of the Campbell's soup ad, "Mmmmgood!" or the strong slurping noise that is common in Japanese culture when sipping tasty soup. Or, the long "Ah-hhhh" we let out after taking a sip of coffee on a rainy morning. Somehow, the sounds we make add to our experience of eating. And then, of course, while eating, we hear comments about how flavorful the food is—"Isn't this cake the best you've ever tasted?" "I've never had a peach so juicy!" Our auditory input certainly adds to our experience of eating. Kimberly notices that she gets great satisfaction from comments given to her about the pumpkin pie that she makes every Thanksgiving. These words feed her in a nourishing way, in much the same way as the pumpkin pie gives delight to her family members.

The dynamic interface of the nose, lips, mouth, and tongue furnishes us with a hotbed of sensory receptors that all work together to give us immediate feedback. Once we smell food, salivation starts to kick in, and digestive juices start to squirt into the stomach. Our nose and tongue work in tandem. Without smell, we lose our ability to taste food. George was born without the ability to smell, so he was unable to taste food. For him, eating had become much more about the textures of food. He liked steak because of the chewy texture and the feeling of fullness he had after eating it. Perhaps you have experienced this sensation temporarily when you had a cold. Think of how having a stuffy nose made eating less enjoyable and how tasty foods became when you felt better!

For some individuals, the texture of foods even more than the taste can be the main factor influencing their choice of food. For Mark, hardboiled eggs have a rubbery texture that makes him cringe; however, scrambled or eggs prepared over-easy are acceptable. Similarly, many people who do not grow up eating tofu find that it has a texture that takes getting used to. Our aversion or particularities around food texture can be traced back to our throat chakra.

THROAT CHAKRA FOODS AND EATING HEALING PLAN

Chew Food

I have heard many a parent in a restaurant gently reprimanding his children to slow down and "*chew* their food." When we are busy, it is easy to slip into the mode of gulping our food down to save time. Some of us even like to drink our food, and have high-protein shakes for convenience. However, there are different physiological and energetic responses to chewing versus swallowing our food. When we chew food, we unlock its messages gradually. We enter into a greater, more complex relationship with the food in its natural state, as it has not been altered. We read the history and travels of a food better when we chew it. On the other hand, when we drink food, such as blending a fruit smoothie, we get different messages. The signals from the food are quickly assimilated into our physiology. The energetic matrix of a food is altered if we puree, blend, or liquefy it. This change isn't necessarily detrimental. It is simply a different translation of what the food has in store for us. As a comparison, think of a family and their genetic connection with each other. Some people in the family resemble one another. There is a familiar tone when they are gathered. However, if nonfamily guests were brought into this arrangement, the exchanges between the family members may be altered. Maybe Uncle Tom would be livelier or tell more jokes. Perhaps young Suzie would have a new playmate and leave her younger sister behind. Thus, patterns change. When two or more ingredients come together to form a new food matrix, a new energy results.

How one eats says volumes about her throat chakra. Guzzling and gulping foods that are meant to be chewed is indicative of some throat chakra issues about being true to ourselves. We do not take the time to look to our depths. When we eat quickly without chewing with consciousness, it is like shortcutting to the *Reader's Digest* version of eating. We are shortchanging ourselves of the richness of the eating experience. Chances are that eating so quickly will only make us hungry later, as we are not fully gathering the authenticity of the eating experience. As a result, the body will search for more satisfying experiences. Also, we may develop indigestion followed by fatigue, because we will be leaving the solar plexus chakra to do all the work. If we go for a period of time only drinking food, a tendency to crave chewing finally develops. Breaking food apart into smaller bits helps our solar plexus chakra to transform these bits into powerful energy. For example, the mouth is where the digestive process starts, and much of our starch digestion occurs here. We can help the throat, heart, and solar plexus chakras work better together when the throat chakra takes on its responsibility to chew food adequately.

Synchronize Eating with Other Throat Chakra Activity

Since the throat chakra area is loaded with all types of activity—talking, tasting, hearing, chewing, breathing, and swallowing—we need to ensure that these activities are synchronized in a way that is balanced. When we take in big gulps of food and swallow in conjunction with breathing erratically, we develop hiccups. You may have heard the phrase, "Don't talk with your mouth full." If we are busy talking and listening, we may not be able to focus on tasting or chewing our food thoroughly enough. So, the essence of synchronizing is to establish a rhythm. No chewing while talking or swallowing, and connecting our breath to our bites of food is a good place to start.

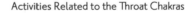

Activities Related to the Throat Chakras

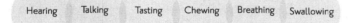

Hearing Talking Tasting Chewing Breathing Swallowing

Once we place our awareness in the proper coordination of activities while we are eating, our throat chakra will fall right into balance and our food will be led into the transformative process. It is when we are busy or not paying attention that we can slip out of this rhythm.

Eat Authentically, Respectfully

The heart chakra is largely about gratitude, and as it relates to food and eating, giving thanks for a meal. The throat chakra voices the gratitude of the heart chakra through words, prayers, and intentions. Its vibration is enhanced in the presence of eating authentically and with respect for the plants and animals that are being eaten, and also for the people, including yourself, that you are eating with. When we eat with respect, we become respect-able: we are able to be respected as well. The reverence and dignity we have for nature and the provision of foods manifests into other areas of our lives. Some traditions honor respectful eating practices by eating foods blessed by a spiritual person or by eating only certain foods on designated days.

Eat in Harmony with Your Metabolism

Everybody has their own rhythm. I often hear, "I am not a morning person" offered as a rationale for not eating breakfast. Others will comment that they have a unique time of the day that they usually get hungry. Yes, the body is quite adaptable. However, it is also meaningful to honor your body's circadian rhythm and your eating patterns. You will have to discern whether you have these patterns due to living or eating a certain way, such as repeatedly eating high glycemic index sugary foods (see chapter 6) that drain your energy and cause you to eat every couple of hours, or whether your body has this pattern hardwired into it. There are a number of studies on the benefits of breakfast. If I know that someone has difficulty eating breakfast, there are ways to meet in the middle. An example of a mealtime compromise might mean having a small piece of fruit rather than a large vegetable-and-egg scramble.

> The throat chakra voices the gratitude of the heart chakra through words, prayers, and intentions.

Try to step back and observe your body's eating rhythm. Shift your schedule on certain days to see whether the pattern is inherent in you or if it is a function of your lifestyle. By doing so, you are honoring the rhythm and balance of your thyroid gland, which is under the oversight of the throat chakra.

Remember that there exists an association among the root, solar plexus, and throat chakras. One example of how they connect energetically is through the muscles. Muscles, supported by the root chakra, are closely connected to our metabolism. The body's basal metabolic rate, or the amount of energy one burns at rest, is proportional to our muscle mass. When we nourish the root chakra by feeding ourselves healthy protein, like soy protein, we can preserve the bulk and functioning of the muscle. The muscle is one of the tissues that insulin responds to; therefore, having good healthy muscles will benefit glucose and insulin metabolism in the body (a function that connects to the solar plexus chakra). As a result, ensuring healthy muscles by focusing on the root chakra can lead to improvements in the balancing of glucose and insulin in the body, which will influence our metabolism.

Eat High-Quality Foods

At the heart of the throat chakra we have choice. Our small and big choices cause a ripple effect into our lives, the lives of others, and the state of the planet. Imagine watching the movie of your life at some point, seeing the result of all of your choices. Which ones will you be satisfied with? The act of eating implicates the element of choice. When you are confronted with food choices, what factors go into making your choice? Cost? Convenience? Taste? Health? Maybe it varies depending on the moment.

The throat chakra is largely about making the highest choice in every moment. It is about a good, quality decision that is well thought out or well felt. If you have the opportunity to eat organic, do you? Should you? And genetically modified organisms—do these matter to you? You may want to explore these questions for yourself to see where your throat chakra is resonating. There are several layers of high-quality eating. You can explore them in any number of ways. For instance, if health is your guiding light when it comes to food purchases, and if you have a craving for chocolate, perhaps you might think about some high-quality, 70 percent cocoa bar rather than the milk chocolate bar loaded with grams of sugar. In this way, you honor your body's need while presenting it with the most healthful option available. In essence, "you can have your cake, and eat it too"!

Introduce Variety

The throat chakra is experiential and uses the senses to maximize its contact with the external world. Therefore, healing the throat chakra through foods involves getting a variety of foods in the diet. Most people settle into what I refer to as "eating ruts," or established eating patterns, which can be a numbing experience. After awhile, it becomes comfortable and doesn't require much thought to eat, and in the long run, eating becomes a lackluster activity and the throat chakra becomes deadened. When we eat the same food(s) all the time, there is also a greater chance of developing a food sensitivity or allergy. This is the body's protective mechanism of encouraging stability (anchored in the root chakra) through variety (the goal of the throat chakra).

What brings a throat chakra to life is an assortment of colors, tastes, and smells to soothe it. Presenting it with a palette of options will provide the throat chakra with the ability to both choose and experience. The Ayurvedic approach to eating, with a mixture of hot and cold foods, and spicy, sour, sweet, bitter, and astringent foods all in one meal, is a perfect way to balance the throat chakra with foods.

On the other hand, variety needs to be kept in check. Too much variety may lead to binge eating. Luxurious buffets are known for prompting excessive eating. Provocative research by Hoch and colleagues has shown that the same amount of food spread into twelve small bowls at a party versus three large ones results in more snacking by partygoers. Similarly, Kahn and Wansink revealed through their clever consumer research that just three more colors of M&Ms in a bowl can lead to more munching (an average of forty-three more M&Ms).

Overall, the "right" amount of variety keeps our throat chakra satisfied and prevents us from overeating (too much variety) and from developing food sensitivities and allergies (too little variety).

FOODS FOR COMMUNICATION AND TRUTH

The five-pointed star is the ideal image symbolizing foods for the throat chakra, as it represents the hub of the complexity of the five senses: smell, hearing, tasting, seeing (governed by its neighbor, the third eye chakra), and touch (under the embrace of the lower heart chakra). The five points speak to the five tastes of food that we are capable of sensing with our tongue: salty, sweet, bitter, sour, and savory. The star shines forth its brilliance—it resonates with crystalline communication. These facets of our bodies show us the way and truth. In much the same way, the energy of our throat chakra leads us to the path of discovering our inner truth.

Additionally, foods that balance the throat chakra are usually foods that bridge the elemental nature of foods. As discussed in previous chapters, each of the chakras up to the heart chakra has an element associated with it: the root chakra symbolizes earth; sacral chakra, water; solar plexus chakra, fire; and heart chakra, air. The throat chakra is ethereal in nature. Its job is to link together the elements of the lower chakras and to bring them together within foods.

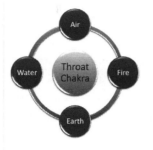

Sea Plants (Water-Earth)
Plants derived from the sea, like nori, agar, dulse, hijiki, arame, and kelp, are excellent sources of nourishment for the throat chakra. Symbolically, these plants represent the earth element, but they have the ability to live in water. Therefore, they beautifully illustrate the earth-water connection, or strengthening the bond between the root and sacral chakras. Through these precious sea sources, the throat chakra can act as an anchor to our lower chakras.

Many people in Western society aren't familiar with edible sea plants other than perhaps the pressed sheet of nori that sushi is rolled in. However, in other countries, particularly Japan, sea plants are a staple of the diet. These magnificent plants are rich in minerals from the sea, including iodine, which is a nutrient that plays a role in proper functioning of the thyroid gland. Iodine is part of the thyroid hormones that help regulate our metabolism. Goiter, or an enlargement of the thyroid gland in the throat, develops when we do not have enough iodine in our diet. In this condition, the throat chakra has to overcompensate, and it extends in an unhealthy way.

Soups (Earth-Water)
Soups represent the fusion between an earth-based food and the element of water. Again, this food is another harmonious mix for blending and stabilizing the root and sacral chakras. Hot and cold soups are wholesome combinations

that support the throat chakra. Most times, soups contrast to ready-to-drink high-calorie beverages in that they take time to eat. Usually, they are eaten one spoonful or sip at a time, creating harmony in the throat chakra. Since the particulates are in a digestible form, there is little energy expended from the throat and solar plexus chakras.

Sauces (Earth-Water)

In much the same way as soups, sauces represent the same earth-water amalgam. Sauces are seen as toppings for main or side dishes. We do not eat sauces as a meal. Rather, they provide a flavorful coating to dishes. Their ability to add flavor to weave foods together in a unifying way is symbolic of the throat chakra. In a similar fashion, the throat chakra's focus is on maximizing the multitude of flavors and on connecting the other chakras together.

Juices (Water-Earth)

Juices are a superb medium that connects throat, solar plexus, and sacral chakras. If the juices are made from green vegetables, the heart chakra can also be incorporated into part of this network. If comprised of red fruits, the root chakra would join the chakra connection circuit. Juices act to moisten and bring the throat chakra to life. However, if they are consumed too regularly, they could create too much energy in the throat chakra, ultimately resulting in an imbalance in the solar plexus chakra. The increased intake of simple sugars could disturb the fine-tuning of blood sugar under the direction of the solar plexus.

Ethnic Foods

As a fun exercise, I like to have clients explore ethnic foods of their own heritage. Some people are used to eating foods of their native culture; I tell them to explore the origin of those foods and meals. Many people are fascinated with what they find. It forces them to talk to their tribe about the history of their meals. This activity resonates well with strengthening the root and throat chakras together.

At first mention of this task, Carol was a bit apprehensive, as she was choosing to eat raw food and thought that most ethnic foods involved cooking. However, when she took the time to go to some Asian grocery stores, she found some delightful curious foods like lychees. She enjoyed the perfume-like taste of the lychee flesh and decided to incorporate it into her food selection.

Sometimes we stay within our comfort zone with foods. Eating ethnic foods allows us to bring a stream of variety into our habitual world and to experience the truth of eating within other cultures. When we eat these foods, we connect with the people and the culture where this food is eaten and grown. We tap into a huge reservoir of knowledge and experience that we may not otherwise have.

Fruits

Since the throat chakra is the hub of senses and responds quickly to food's physical properties, the throat chakra is sensitive to certain fruits. High-water fruits like watermelon, cucumber, cantaloupe, and grapes can serve the throat chakra by providing sufficient moisture to open this energetic center to make it receptive to and comfortable with speaking the truth. Conversely, astringent or sour fruits like lemon, lime, and kiwi activate the throat chakra to dispel nontruths.

Blue-Colored Foods

Where are all the blue foods? Isn't that a curious question? Interestingly enough, there exist no foods in their natural state that vibrate to the frequency of a sky blue color. Since the throat chakra is already dense with a number of sensory and energetic receptors, it does not need the added stimulus of color to impact it. Dark blue and purple pigments primarily affect the third eye chakra rather than the throat chakra and are addressed in chapter 9 on the third eye chakra.

AFFIRMATIONS TO HEAL THE THROAT CHAKRA

Affirmations are helpful tools that assist us in changing core belief patterns. By writing these words or by saying them on a daily basis, we infuse our subconscious with new patterns. As we continue to make them a part of our surroundings, so will they become part of who we are. Make up your own as you see appropriate. Here are some to get you started.

- *I eat in harmony with my environment.*
- *I chew food with consciousness.*
- *I communicate with myself about my food needs.*
- *I celebrate the diversity of ethnic foods.*
- *My food choices reflect my authenticity.*
- *My meals synergize the connection between my chakras.*

FOOD AND EATING ACTIVITIES
TO BALANCE THE THROAT CHAKRA

- Try the simple practice of chewing your food carefully and slowly until it becomes liquid in your mouth. Focus on creating an abundance of saliva in your mouth, thinking of it as liquid transformative juice. With each bite, see what messages the food is giving you. What insight do you receive? You can also make this an active exercise by infusing messages into every bite of food.
- Allow yourself to listen to the messages of food. Pick a food that you feel drawn to and create a journal dialogue with it.
- Visit an ethnic grocery store and pick one new food to try.
- The throat chakra is responsible for the integration of many levels of information. How is food a metaphor for you in your life? How can it be looked at from a symbolic perspective?
- Where do you lack respect for yourself and become inauthentic in your eating habits? Create a statement of gratitude that is simple to remember. For example, "I give thanks to the miracle of nourishment."
- The next time you are eating with others, observe the balance you have between talking, chewing, and breathing. Are they synchronized? If not, focus on anchoring yourself in your breath and chew in the breathing rhythm.
- Pay attention to the importance of your sense of smell when eating. Does smell add to your experience of eating?
- Note language used around food. How do you express your hunger with words? Your feelings of satisfaction with eating? What words are used on food packaging of foods you eat? Are those messages you choose for your life?

EATING PLAN TO SUPPORT THE THROAT CHAKRA

Choose meals from each of these meal categories in order to complete your throat chakra needs.

Breakfast Options

Smoothies (earth-water)
Mango lassi
Red Whirl Smoothie**
Swiss muesli (ethnic dish)
Fresh juices (water-earth)
Juicy fruits: watermelon, mango, peach

Lunch Options

Chicken tamale with guacamole (ethnic dish)
Kelp soup (sea plant)
Vegetarian Nori Rolls* (sea plant)
Miso soup with Sea-Slaw* (sea plant)

Dinner Options

East Indian meal composed of a variety of tastes (salty, sour, sweet,
    bitter)
Middle Eastern meal of couscous, radishes, kebobs (ethnic meal)
Vegetables with Balsamic Vinegar-Peach Sauce*
Asian Miso-Dulse Soup*

---

* Indicates recipe at back of book

** See root chakra recipes

CHAPTER 9

FOODS FOR INTUITION AND IMAGINATION

Feeding the Third Eye Chakra

*Be curious always, for knowledge
will not acquire you; you must acquire it.*
—SUDIE BACK

Perception • Insight • Wisdom • Dreams •
Psychic Energy • Visualization • Concentration •
Imagination • Self-Realization • Moods • Sleep

TINA: SPIRALING INTO ANOTHER WORLD

Tina finds herself waking up at night, plagued by nightmares. In the mornings, she feels scattered and clumsy due to lack of sleep. Her friends describe her as a "complex" person, and her brother calls her "moody." He says that she is like a woman "who wears a thousand faces" because her disposition is always changing. Although she is unable to spend much time with it, Tina feels best when she

**The third eye
chakra gives us
the ability to align
ourselves with our
inner knowing.**

is expressing herself through her art. If she doesn't paint, she feels like a different person: her imagination takes her over, causing her inner fantasy life to collide with her practical everyday life. As a result, she experiences much chaos in her dealings with people and situations. She easily finds herself overwhelmed with life, and describes it as "sensory overload." Sometimes lights, noise, and color fill her mind, and she is unable to function clearly.

When in the presence of others, she will see images of a particular person in the group flash in front of her. When she sees these images, she imagines impressions about the situation that may change her mood rapidly. Tina recognizes her quick shift in behavior but feels as though she can do nothing about it.

Tina's third eye chakra is not well balanced in that she is unable to mesh together all the dimensions of reality that are presented to her. As a result, she cannot function in a "normal" way on a day-to-day basis. Without a firm division of worlds in place, she mixes them together, causing confusion and chaos. Tina's third eye chakra is in high gear, giving her vivid dreams, an overactive imagination, and an uncontrollable flux of psychic activity. She becomes paralyzed by the influx of information coming in from the outside, like visual stimuli, or conjured from the realm of her internal landscape. Individuals like Tina with third eye complexity appear to be moody because they are responding to the stimuli they are constantly receiving. They lean toward adopting the attitude that life is caving in on them, causing them to lose control. At some point, they lose internal sight of who they are and their Divine mission.

These individuals can be overanalytical, thinking situations into mush. The more they think about a situation, the more they lose sight of their direction and ultimate decision. They second-guess themselves and fill themselves with doubt. Others may take on tendencies of being "obsessive-compulsive." These individuals are so bombarded with their thoughts that they have to find a way to control the situation. Therefore, their effort becomes one of a controlling nature, as this is the only way that they feel they will not go "insane" in their lives.

Depression is another feature of an imbalance at the third eye chakra. The seeds of depression can originate in the heart chakra and ultimately affect the third eye chakra or they can stem from not being open to the third eye chakra. When this is closed down, the neurotransmitter network is impaired, leading to altered behavior, memory, cognition, and even more broadly into personality.

THE THIRD EYE CHAKRA: INSIGHT

UNHEALTHY THIRD EYE CHAKRA INDICATIONS

Tina displays one manifestation of an imbalance in the third eye chakra region. If you have issues to address in your third eye chakra, you might answer "Yes" to the following questions:

* Do you find that you often ruminate or think back over and over on situations?
* Would the people who know you well say you are overanalytical?
* Have you had or do you have issues with addictions, particularly to drugs or alcohol?
* Do you often feel that your mind has a "life of its own"?
* Do you tend to be erratic in your behavior?
* Do you have an active imagination?
* Have you had visions or dreams that have come true?
* Do you have nightmares often?
* Are you obsessive-compulsive?
* Do you frequently crave chocolate?
* Do you feel that your thinking is blocked?
* Do you feel cut off from your internal vision and life purpose?
* Do you rarely dream or remember your dreams?
* Is your mind often "blank," unable to respond appropriately to decisions?
* Do you find yourself sleeping an excessive amount compared to other people?
* Do you or have you suffered from depression?
* Do you feel that you are a victim of your life experience?
* Do you find that you need external stimulants (for example, caffeine) to keep you going?

HEALTHY THIRD EYE CHAKRA BEHAVIOR

The third eye chakra is probably the most magical, mystical chakra, as it is seen as the portal to enlightenment for many cultures and religions. It is located in the center of the forehead and extends inward to the corresponding space inside the head. Essentially, it serves as the control board of our spiritual, mental, emotional, and physical being. It provides insight into the hardwiring of who we truly are and the means for us to get to our truth. The third eye chakra, when open to its full potential, has the ability to help us separate truth from illusion. Simply put, it endows us with a beacon of insight in our panoramic experience of life from a place of wisdom and truth.

When opened fully, this chakra gives us the tools of awareness of ourselves as spiritual beings and of wisdom. It can open our awareness into that of other worlds and can expose us to a deep knowing of who we are and what our path entails. A healthy, functioning third eye chakra will be able to follow our internal visions and dreams, knowing that they are being Divinely guided and inspired. When our life is aligned with our intuition, our thoughts and actions will be resolute. There will be no room for second-guessing.

The third eye chakra gives us the ability to align ourselves with our inner knowing of what nurtures us on many levels. Individuals with well-developed third eye chakras are able to step into a "psychic" knowing for themselves and others. If the chakra is vibrating at an accelerated frequency, they open up to psychic information that transcends time and space, a doorway to rich possibilities and discernment. If likened to a person, the third eye chakra would be a wise parent or a being with royal stature. Whereas the heart may be seen as the emotional sovereign, the third eye can be likened to the sovereignty of insight.

This center is most often first engaged whenever our mind is involved: when we meditate, pray, or dream. Mind-centering activities will unlock this chakra, causing it to connect us immediately with Spirit. Ancient East Indian practices speak to the release of creative, kundalini energy from the root chakra and its journey up the spine to infuse the mind, or the third eye chakra, for enhanced insight. Since this chakra underlies the mind, brain, and thoughts, it is responsible for much mental activity and for manifesting our thoughts and vision. Dreams are important messengers to those with a healthy third eye chakra. They will be in touch with their inner landscape through their dreams and turn these signs into valuable, meaningful truths to apply to their waking life.

When activated, the third eye chakra is the all-knowing, all-seeing chakra and is quite different from the other chakras in that it is our passage to Spirit. Whereas the throat chakra speaks to the interplay of our choices on Earth, our will, and Divine Will, the third eye chakra is the landscape of our dreams and our higher knowing and wisdom. It is much more ethereal than the other chakras that have been discussed. The third eye chakra allows us to abandon our need to control and to dive head on into whatever we are presented with, with utmost confidence that it is the best possible situation for us. The throat chakra may present us with a crossroads or with potential choices for a particular situation, but the third eye glows with the truth of recognizing that whatever happens is the only thing that could have happened.

THE FOUR WAYS OF "SEEING"

The throat chakra provides us with senses to take in messages from the physical realm. The tongue can taste food, and this experience nourishes us. The third eye chakra connects to the portals of the throat chakra, especially the eyes, which link primarily to the third eye chakra, to gift us with nonphysical messages. These messages may be divined through to us from our highest self, angels, guides, avatars, or whoever else is looking after us. The information can reflect what is to come or what has already happened. Time makes no difference for these psychic senses—clairvoyance (seeing insightful images), clairsentience (feeling insight), clairaudience (hearing insight), and what I like to call "clair-olfactance" (smelling insight)—because they operate in the realm of timelessness. We can be strong in one or more of these psychic senses.

> **The third eye glows with the truth of recognizing that whatever happens is the only thing that could have happened.**

Clairvoyance is receiving inner and Divine knowing through the gift of sight. Gayle describes clairvoyance: "I was sitting at the stoplight in traffic, and before me, I had this vision of a truck colliding head-on with a smaller vehicle in the intersection. The next day I was reading the paper and saw that an accident had occurred at that intersection later that day." Clairsentience simply refers to a "knowing." There is no particular sense involved, but it is information you recognize at a deep level, rather "matter-of-fact." It's an experience where you can shrug your shoulders and say, "I just know that to be true." Clairaudience, or hearing insight, is often experienced by those with a strong throat chakra, since it's the throat chakra that connects with the ears. Josh relays his experience: "I was walking through a department store and I heard a voice that told me to turn left rather than right. About ten feet further, I ran into my childhood friend that I hadn't seen in years!" The third eye chakra points us in the direction that there are no coincidences. Every action, word, and thought are purposefully intended and guided.

Like clairaudience, "clair-olfactance" involves the throat chakra energy, since it focuses on the nose and sense of smell. You can walk through a space and, all of a sudden, you smell a distinct scent rather intensely. This aroma may trigger your third chakra synapses to connect with other information that you need to know. For example, Sarah became very distraught at a team meeting. She excused herself and walked out of the room. Immediately, she was overcome with the smell of roses, even though no roses were in sight. The roses reminded her of her grandmother, who was always supportive and loving. After a couple of minutes of being connected with her loving grandmother's energy by smelling roses, she decided to return to the meeting in a relaxed state, with a smile on her face.

ILLUSION

Whereas Christ connects with heart chakra energy, Buddha lives within the third eye chakra. Buddhism focuses on reining in the mind through meditative practices. Controlling our thoughts rather than allowing them to control us is essential for the third eye chakra. Because of the infinite power that we receive through this chakra, we can easily become overwhelmed. However, when we are able to watch our thoughts like clouds, allowing them to flow through us rather than sticking to us like cotton candy, we feel healthier and free. We release ourselves from being a prisoner of our minds.

Meditation is a tool by which we can liberate ourselves from the earth illusion. As Christ commented, "Be in the world, but not of it." The third eye chakra helps us to do just this, and in our everyday life to separate fact from fiction. It is helpful to view life as a movie, watching it unfold in front of you, rather than becoming attached and stuck.

The Buddhist principle speaks to cultivating "loving detachment." Again, the heart chakra and third eye chakra share close circuitry. The heart chakra embodies emotional wisdom and maturity. The third eye chakra takes this embodiment one step further into "loving detachment" by helping us to put the situation into larger perspective. Work within the heart chakra is like peering into the trees, whereas the third eye chakra zooms out to look at the expanse of the forest. Practicing loving detachment is an excellent exercise for those who get swallowed up in the depths of their minds and who stay stuck in emotional grooves from the past. With our third eye chakra, we have the ability to see life as an illusion. And, when we synchronize this perspective with that of the throat chakra by surrendering to Divine will, we reside in blissful balance.

MICROCOSM VERSUS MACROCOSM

As mentioned, the third eye chakra is very good at giving us perception and objectivity. It allows us to see the dimensions embedded in all living beings: the microcosms within the macrocosms, and vice versa. The microcosm of our cells make up the macrocosm of our being. The microcosm of all people makes up the macrocosm of the Earth. We vacillate within the spiral of our smallness and largeness at all times. We have access to becoming expansive and opening ourselves up to the collective consciousness, or the universal mind, to channel information for our everyday lives. Many Indian yogis have described being able to be "in two places at once": their spiritual essence connects to this immense consciousness layer and their physical body stays within the earthly existence.

Expanding ourselves in this direction helps us to attain a state of "self-realization," or the tip of Maslow's hierarchical pyramid. In this state, we recognize and accept our separation and our oneness with all that is. The third eye chakra embraces opposites, similar to the sacral chakra, but on a much larger scale.

Core Issues Associated with the Third Eye Chakra
- Aligning with Divine guidance
- Balancing one's personality to prevent moodiness and volatility
- Being able to process thoughts within the realm of experience
- Being decisive
- Following one's dreams
- Separating truth from illusion
- Trust in one's ability
- Understanding one's personal truth

THE NATURE OF THE INTUITION VIBRATION

Whereas the throat chakra focuses on the freedom of the light blue sky that engulfs Earth, the third eye chakra looks beyond our immediate atmosphere and turns toward the indigo-colored universe, beyond the realm of Earth's vision, into that of other worlds and planetary existence. The third eye chakra resonates with the blanket of the star-speckled universe that envelops us and gives us a sense of perspective and trust that we are a part of a larger macrocosm with a perfect design and plan. The third eye chakra asks us to trust that our internal wisdom and knowing will lead the way.

Readings of this center will often be multidimensional and more psychedelic than earthy. Often, it will present itself as a journey or a spiraling vortex of colors.

PHYSIOLOGY OF THE THIRD EYE CHAKRA

The third eye chakra encompasses many physical and nonphysical workings of the being. Physically, the third eye chakra relates to the eyes, the forehead, and the pineal gland, which controls the clockwork of our secretions and rhythms. The third eye chakra is the center that balances and integrates hormones in the body. It oversees the brain and thoughts and therefore is directly linked with the production of and workings of our neurotransmitters, such as serotonin and dopamine. Through this connection, the third eye is vastly responsible for moods and the projected personality of the self.

Anatomy Associated with the Third Eye Chakra

- Brain
- Eyebrows
- Eyes
- Forehead
- Neurotransmitters
- Pineal gland
- Regulation of hormone function

THE RELATIONSHIP OF INTUITION AND IMAGINATION TO FOODS AND EATING

THIRD EYE CHAKRA FOOD AND EATING HEALING PLAN

Eat Intuitively

In chapter 4, on the root chakra, we discussed questioning the body on its food needs, an active process designed to help us to better read and dialogue with our physiology. Intuitive eating can be both an active and a passive process. Sometimes we feel strongly at the gut level that we need to eat certain foods. Perhaps we are reading a book and, all of a sudden, without any association to what we were reading, we have a strong feeling that our body would do well with some steamed spinach. During and after eating the spinach, there is a sense of alignment within our being. We may feel more resonant, more vibrant. There are other times when you can simply intuit what you need to eat. Maybe you are looking over a restaurant menu with a variety of choices, wondering what to order. You can certainly ask your body what it needs and begin that conversation. Alternately, you can focus on your third eye and ask to be guided to the dish on the menu that would be in congruence with your highest self. You may be surprised by what you are led to eat! Flexing your intuitive muscle with respect to eating is an important skill to develop. Some people feel doubt about the information they may receive; however, the more we honor the insight coming forth, the more readily it will come and the more we will start to trust it. We must practice, like many other activities!

When we are not in sync with the intuition generated by our third eye chakra, we may resort to "analysis paralysis" when it comes to eating. Overintellectualizing eating by reducing it to calories or grams of macronutrients, crafting habits about how we eat and allowing the noisy obsessive-compulsive part of us take over the foods we choose squelches our intuitive wisdom. Rather than have your third eye be boxed in by the structure of what and how you are eating (which can lead to a certain degree of insanity!), embrace the deep resounding intuition spiraling from your third eye chakra.

Understand Addictions to Food

Some individuals may feel that they are addicted to eating certain foods. This addiction surpasses the occasional craving and takes a strong hold on our being. It becomes the commander of our third eye chakra. A common food addiction is sugar-containing foods, as they impart a temporary sense of power (in the solar plexus chakra) and an energy surge to send our neuron synapses firing in all directions (in the third eye chakra). Maybe there is a specific food item that we do not feel like we can mentally escape from—chocolate is a popular one.

I have witnessed several fascinating discoveries around food addictions, from childhood memories to a call for more of something in their lives. For example, one person's intense draw to ice cream was connected to her innate loneliness. When she was a child, she would go with children in the neighborhood in the summertime to the local ice cream shop. It made her summers memorable. Now, as an adult, she felt isolated and was, on a subconscious level, eating the ice cream as a way to resurrect the memory of community and friendship. She had no idea of this relationship between the two until she did this activity.

Laddering Techniques to Access the Root of Food Addictions

One way to uncover our subconscious connection to a food addiction is by mining the landscape of the third eye chakra. When we understand our deeper tie to the food, we can more easily overcome the addiction.

To do this technique effectively, work with someone you trust. Have this person guide the process by saying the name of the food that you are addicted to over and over again, usually for about twenty times. Every time you hear the word, say the first word that comes to your mind and have the other person write it down. Continue in successive fashion, very quickly, without judgment. At the end of the exercise, you will have twenty words to work with to find a pattern in or to create a story from.

It helps to have your eyes closed when doing this exercise so that you can focus within and be free of any external distraction. The person guiding you through the exercise should only be writing down your responses and not commenting on them. If you find that after ten times of responding, your mind is blank and nothing comes forth, sit until a word, feeling, or thought arises. When we give ourselves time by being patient, the third eye chakra reveals its mystery.

Nourish the Brain and Mood

The third eye chakra shows us that there is a distinct relationship between food and mood: our foods can influence our moods and our moods can certainly drive our food choices. Food has a powerful effect on our psychology, or our third eye chakra. You have most likely heard of the connection between sugar and hyperactivity in children. The brain prefers to use glucose as a source of fuel. When it is inundated with sugar, it has lots of energy to put out. Energetically, the brain may feel like it has been overloaded, saturated with the substance.

Conversely, eating turkey or drinking warm milk may cause you to feel sleepy. As you remember from the root chakra chapter, these foods are highly grounding. They are going to slow our body's reactions and stabilize us. Similarly, these foods will cause our brain chemistry to change. Turkey contains the amino acid tryptophan, which is the building block for serotonin, the neurotransmitter in the brain that gives us that "feel good," and even dissociated, sensation.

On the other hand, our moods may compel us to eat a certain way. As we discussed in the sacral chakra chapter (chapter 5), if we are not feeling our emotions, we can bury them into food and eating. Moods act similarly to emotions. Whereas emotions are raw and short-lived, moods slip over us like a sheath. We take on a certain tone that encompasses emotional response along with the psychic energy of the whole being. Just like the heart chakra reaches out several feet within its vicinity to pick up emotional input, the third eye chakra is an antenna for universal consciousness. This consciousness gets wrapped up into our mood. Our moods may tell us to eat chocolate for days on end. Or maybe we are "in the mood" for lemon sorbet.

The sacral chakra is intimately connected to both the heart and third eye chakras. The fats and oils discussed in the sacral chakra chapter are large constituents of brain matter. Our thoughts and behavior are strongly governed by the amount of essential fats in our brain. When we do not have enough emotional flow coming through our sacral chakra, our heart and third eye chakra are prone to collapse. For the third eye chakra, this state manifests as depression. Eating healthy fats can encourage more flow in the body, from the sacral chakra up to the third eye, releasing us from depression.

> **Emotions are raw and short-lived; moods slip over us like a sheath.**

Eat to Enhance Concentration

Concentration, which falls under the auspices of the third eye chakra, can be improved significantly by eating. When we have to study for a test, or to complete a physical task, our third eye chakra is active. Food provides the energy that we need to feed this center so that we can maintain our focus. Those with attention deficient disorder, commonly referred to as ADD, have a revved third eye chakra. Refraining from eating foods that stimulate the third eye chakra may be beneficial for these individuals, allowing them to concentrate.

Eat for the Planet

The third eye chakra extends us beyond our individual needs to examine consciousness at large. Sometimes we get lost in the microcosm of our own mind or body and forget that we connect with other forms of life at our core. The way that we choose to eat ultimately affects the entire magnitude of every living organism. Thus, your third eye chakra asks you: How are you eating to support the greater whole, which includes you? Are you eating in such a way to support life on planet Earth? Of the many opportunities we have on a daily basis to interact with foods and eating, how many of those are we making meaningful for the human race, the animal kingdom, and the plant families? The third eye chakra sparks us to actively involve ourselves in collective consciousness. By being aware of our food choices, we honor the call of the third eye chakra to serve the planet.

Eat for Improved Sleep

Moving into the dark, nighttime hours resonates with the third eye chakra more than any other chakra. When we overtax our mind, we may use food to unwind it, particularly after a long day at work. Many people engage in uncontrollable nighttime snacking that can throw off their third eye chakra balance, including their sleep pattern, circadian rhythm, and delicate hormone cycles. Our quality and quantity of sleep can be improved by shifting our eating cycles into a rhythm that works for us. Most people sleep soundly when they do not eat close to bedtime. Not eating two to three hours before bedtime usually works well. If we eat right before we go to sleep, our third eye chakra may remain too active, keeping us unsettled throughout the night. On the other hand, having a light protein snack right before bedtime may help give individuals with a third eye chakra imbalance (affecting other chakras like root and solar plexus) a more deep, grounded quality of sleep.

You may find that eating closer to bedtime or eating certain foods in the evening influences the quality and intensity of your dreams. Eating foods high in sugar or caffeine in the evening puts the third eye chakra into overdrive during the sleeping hours, creating vivid dreams and, in some people, even nightmares. For restful dreams, curtail nighttime eating.

FOODS FOR INTUITION AND IMAGINATION

Foods for intuition and imagination are symbolized by the spiral. The spiral is a long-recognized archetype for cycles, such as the emerging and ending of a new day and the cycle of life-death-rebirth. Much of life's lessons are learned in a spiral fashion—we are the same person, but revisit the same situation time and time again. At each time that we visit it, we have a new perception because the fabric of our being has been altered to give us fresh eyes. The third eye chakra assists us in opening up to new perceptions on foods. Foods that resonate with this center unlock our insight in a rhythmic manner.

As we clarified in chapter 8, on the throat chakra, there will be less of a connection with a physical substance like food in chakras like the third eye, since these are the less Earthbound parts of ourselves. Often, there is some other characteristic about the food that is symbolic for the chakra. For example, foods that stimulate and help to balance the excesses of a higher chakra are those of a potent nature. They are usually more intense, concentrated foods that create a dramatic physiological response using only a small amount. Of course, with the third eye chakra and its obsessive nature, the response of these foods in the body may be so overwhelming that they could become dizzying (back to the spiral) and addictive (going 'round and 'round).

Caffeine

Caffeine feeds the third eye chakra and can lead to mood-altering effects. If you think about the foods that contain caffeine, such as coffee, black and green teas, and chocolate, you know that these foods have a strong charge in our society. Depending on the individual, a certain quantity of caffeine may be useful in stimulating the third chakra. In nonusers or occasional users of caffeine, low doses (less than 200 mg) can produce a heightened sense of awareness and well-being. However, repeated use may result in ongoing dependency.

When we are constantly stimulating our third eye chakra, we create a *need* for the stimulation. When we ingest foods consistently and without consciousness, there is the risk that we may become attached to them. They can become addictive and even result in low-level withdrawal symptoms, like tiredness in the mornings. The third eye chakra is one of the main centers that activates when someone has an addiction, no matter what the substance. With continued use, caffeine engages the third eye chakra to spin at an increased rate, creating an imbalance in the other chakra systems. Soon after, we may realize that we are frenetic and unable to concentrate on tasks and simple activities due to the overactive busyness of the mind. In other words, addictive foods may move us into a realm that we are not prepared for.

When people attempt to eliminate coffee from the body for one day or in the course of an elimination diet, they immediately start to develop symptoms that can be quite severe. The body releases caffeine in much the same way as a drug: the body shakes, sweats, aches, and usually headaches are brought on that last for days, depending on how long and how much caffeine had been ingested over time. On the chakra level, the third eye is releasing its hold on the altered reality created by the caffeine itself. Since the physical body moves more slowly than the other layers of our selves, the physical body takes a noticeable hit. It shifts back to its original state. Most people notice that once they have given up the need for caffeine, they feel less anxious. When the third eye chakra is activated, the energy gets sent to the other chakras it is networked with, which in this case, is the heart chakra.

On the flip side, caffeine-containing foods can be quite conducive to quick thinking and mental organization when used in their proper context. Remember that it is key to question what your body needs on a daily basis so that you will provide it with what it needs for its activities.

Chocolate

There is probably no other food that connects to the third eye chakra more potently than chocolate. If someone craves chocolate, this is a direct indication that they have some third eye chakra activity happening. Specifically, individuals who deplete their third eye chakra's reserves by overthinking or by taxing their psychic skill may find that they crave chocolate. Chocolate's vibration replenishes and stimulates a drained third eye chakra. In certain countries, like the United States, chocolate is a coveted item; in other countries, like Brazil, chocolate is not as desired and craved, suggesting that there are cultural energetic patterns that create specific eating patterns.

Chocolate can change our mood, as it contains several constituents that act as stimulants or that give us the comforting "I'm in love" feeling. It draws us when we are feeling the need for love or the need for intensity, or, in other words, to open our heart and third eye chakras. It is also a food that plays in the arena of the sacral chakra, as it is often used as a means of emotional release. Eating chocolate is used as a bypass for expressing emotion; however, researchers Macdiarmid and Hetherington revealed that eating chocolate for emotional reasons causes only negative emotions.

On a pure food science level, there is much research touting the benefits of chocolate. In addition to the caffeine it contains (see Table 9.1), cocoa in its pure form contains relatively high amounts of antioxidants known as *flavonoids*, which can help to open up our blood vessels. It has been purported by some researchers that due to these compounds, cocoa may be beneficial for the heart, and a small daily intake of dark chocolate can lead to decreased blood pressure. This effect affirms the concept that cocoa stimulates the third eye chakra to open, causing changes in the heart and sacral chakras.

Studies investigating chocolate cravings have shown that no other food really substitutes for a chocolate craving. If someone has a craving for something sweet, usually one or more items can be eaten and that craving satisfied. Not so for a chocolate craving! There is something uniquely different about chocolate. In a study by researchers Michener and Rozin at the University of Pennsylvania, subjects were given capsules containing the therapeutic, healthy actives in chocolate, others were given a white chocolate bar (containing none of the actives that you normally get from eating cocoa), and some others were given a milk chocolate bar. The group given the milk chocolate bar had reduced cravings compared to all the other groups. Therefore, it's not necessarily about the goodies in the chocolate. There is perhaps a combined effect of the sensory input of the chocolate (slightly bittersweet, smooth texture) with the presense of individual constituents that create physiological responses that make people love it.

Spices

As a category, spices work primarily through the third eye chakra and influence the respective chakra centers. Spices are pungent materials, needed only in small amounts to have a strong flavoring effect. Many of these botanicals are so potent that they also have medicinal properties. When spices are used liberally in cooking, they add to the flavorful impact of foods and act to bridge the chakras through their unifying effects. For example, cinnamon has effects on several chakras, with the solar plexus chakra most dramatically affected due to its warming ("fire") effect and its ability to assist in the body's handling of blood sugar. Curry has strong antioxidant activity, and studies show that eating it can help protect the brain. Therefore, curry resonates directly with the third eye chakra. It is stimulatory but also protective.

Table 9.1   Caffeine Content of Common Food Items

	Substance	Serving Size (volume or weight)	Caffeine Content (range)	Caffeine Content (typical)
Coffee	Brewed/Drip	6 oz.	77–150 mg	100 mg
	Instant	6 oz.	20–130 mg	70 mg
	Espresso	1 oz.	30–50 mg	40 mg
	Decaffeinated	6 oz.	2–9 mg	4 mg
Tea	Brewed	6 oz.	30–90 mg	40 mg
	Instant	6 oz.	10–35 mg	30 mg
	Canned or bottled	12 oz.	8–32 mg	20 mg
	Caffeinated soft drinks	12 oz.	22–71 mg	40 mg
Chocolate	Cocoa/Hot chocolate	6 oz.	2–10 mg	7 mg
	Milk chocolate	1.5 oz.	2–10 mg	10 mg
	Dark chocolate	1.5 oz.	5–35 mg	30 mg

Source: Johns Hopkins Medical Center, *www.caffeinedependence.org/caffeine_dependence.html*

Alcohol and Drugs

Any substance that alters our consciousness affects and clouds the third eye chakra. Of course, alcohol and recreational drugs are likely candidates. Individuals who overuse either of these tend to have a thick, mucus-like energy hovering in the third chakra terrain that can cause stagnation in the other areas of the chakra circuit, particularly the crown chakra (severing contact with the Divine) and the throat chakra (giving over sense of truth and authenticity to these conscious-altering vehicles). Eventually, the third eye chakra will be depleted, manifesting as depression and lethargy. In moderate amounts, however, red wine can be balancing for the third eye chakra due to the essence of grapes it contains, resonating to this center's purple vibration.

Spices to Stimulate and Protect the Third Eye Chakra

- Allspice
- Anise
- Basil
- Caraway
- Cardamom
- Chili powder
- Coriander
- Cumin
- Curry
- Dill
- Fennel
- Fenugreek
- Ginger
- Horseradish
- Mint
- Nutmeg
- Pepper
- Sage
- Turmeric
- Wasabi

Purple-Red Foods

Purple foods such as grapes, blueberries, and blackberries contain purplish-colored antioxidants known as *anthocyanidins*. Relative to other antioxidants, these have the greatest "punch" in their ability to quench damaging free radicals. The anthocyanidin family of compounds acts to protect the third eye chakra primary territory of the brain and nervous system from stress injury. Ingesting them will help to nourish the third eye chakra and, more important, will protect it from psychic attack and overwork. The third eye chakra is also nourished by small, intensely flavored reddish fruits such as red currants, raspberries, and pomegranate.

Purple-Red Foods to Nourish the Third Eye Chakra

Vegetables	Fruit
Eggplant	Blackberries
Purple cabbage	Blueberries
Purple kale	Boysenberries
Purple potato	Figs
	Marionberries
	Plums
	Purple grapes
	Raisins

AFFIRMATIONS TO HEAL THE THIRD EYE CHAKRA

Affirmations are helpful tools that assist us in changing core belief patterns. By writing these words or by saying them on a daily basis, we infuse our subconscious with new patterns. As we continue to make them a part of our surroundings, so will they become part of who we are. Make up your own as you see appropriate. Here are some to get you started.

- *Intuition guides my food choices.*
- *Purple foods enhance my inner and outer vision.*
- *I eat to nourish my brain and thinking.*
- *Eating connects me to universal consciousness.*
- *Spices allow my gift of intensity to surface.*
- *Chocolate clears my psychic center.*

FOOD AND EATING ACTIVITIES
TO BALANCE THE THIRD EYE CHAKRA

- Before you start eating, clear your mind by meditating for five minutes. Empty all the thoughts that you choose to release from having influence on the energy of the foods you ingest.
- Create a mantra that you can use to focus and harness your mental energy around your relationship with foods. For example, if you obsess about the quantity of food you eat and find yourself within the thick of condemning thoughts after a meal, reset your third eye chakra with a mantra such as "I eat as much as I need; I eat as much as I need."
- Practice using your intuition to make food choices when you are at the market. What do you hear? What do you see? Are these sense-signals triggers to what you need to be paying attention to?
- Do an experiment to investigate the relationship between foods and your dreams. Note whether you dream about any particular foods. What significance does that food have for you? How do foods you eat change your dreams? For instance, when you eat meat, do you dreams become more vivid? When you eat green vegetables, do you sleep more deeply?
- Are you a victim of analysis-paralysis when it comes to foods? Do you allow your life to be run by "nutrition-by-number," counting up calories, grams of fat? Through journaling, dialogue with the inner nutritional accountant that may live in your third chakra.

- How is your mood affected by foods? Do you feel happy when you eat certain foods? Fatigued and depressed when you eat others? Keep a brief food log of how foods affect your mood before and after you eat them.
- How can you zoom out of your individual eating experience bubble and connect to the expanse of the greater planetary consciousness of eating? What activities can you do to assist others in being fed (for example, participate in a soup kitchen) or to support the sanctity of the food supply (for example, donate to organizations that advocate organic farming practices)? Brainstorm on ideas to help grow the healthy global consciousness of eating, and act on one every season of the year.
- Do you have an addiction to any particular food? What is the root of the addiction? Do the laddering technique to uncover the real reason for the pull to the food.

EATING PLAN TO SUPPORT INTUITION
Of course, it is best to use your own intuition to feed your intuition. However, to get you started with tuning into your third eye chakra, try these meal additions.

Breakfast Options
Ch-Eye Tea*
Grape juice
Fresh mixed berries
Ginger Spice Bread*

Lunch Options
Spicy Thai Meal with Green Tea–Berry Freeze*
Sweet and sour shrimp
Ask your intuition!

After Dinner Options
Choco-ffee Tofu Insight Whip*
Mint tea
Berry Wisdom Seeker Cobbler*

---

* Indicates recipe at back of book

FOODS FOR PURIFICATION AND CLARIFICATION

Feeding the Crown Chakra

*The true way to be humble is not to stoop
until you are smaller than yourself, but to stand at
your real height against some higher nature that will
show you what the real smallness of your greatness is.*
—PHILLIPS BROOKS

Infinite • Awakened • Eternal • Bliss •
Spirituality • Universal Truth • Divine Purpose •
Unity • Highest Self • Absolute • Soul

KEITH: CLOSED TO HIS CROWN

Keith was raised in a very strict religious household. His mother, active in church affairs, had imposed a "house rule" that Keith had to attend services every week with her. Additionally, she volunteered him for several church-related activities without his consent and donated much of the family money to the church, even though they didn't have a great deal. If that weren't enough, she earnestly expressed her wish early on in his life that she would like Keith to become a pastor. By the age of fifteen, Keith felt stifled by his mother's religiosity. At eighteen, he started to develop panic attacks. As a young adult, he withdrew from society by staying inside with the curtains closed, and he even stopped eating for days in a row. His panic attacks continued, and he decided to get help from a psychiatrist. Medications appeared to work temporarily. Keith formed a close bond with a work colleague and told him about his panic attacks and family background. On a daily basis, he began unraveling the wounds of the past to allow enough room in his life to explore his own spirituality.

Keith's mother displayed an exaggerated crown chakra, or a preoccupation with spiritual matters to the degree that it impacts physical life. These individuals are overzealous and even evangelical in their beliefs, wanting others to convert to their belief systems. Often, physical needs such as eating, sleeping, and shelter are overlooked. Frequently, these people are not fully embracing living in their Earth bodies in a healthy way. As a result, there is an imbalance in the physical realm. The overworking of the crown chakra does not necessarily mean that a person is more spiritual or "closer to God." It could simply indicate a frantic, blind following of a belief or a cult.

For Keith, his mother's approach to spirituality backfired. It polarized him to any spiritual beliefs. The crown chakra attracts "misbeliefs" and "disbeliefs." *Misbeliefs* refer to imposed projections of a Higher Power onto another person without that person's consent. These misbeliefs store within the crown chakra and act as a filter for any messages or Divine inspiration coming through. With Keith, he may have taken on the perception that God requires time in church and in service activities and becomes angry and vengeful if these requirements are not met. As a result of this misbelief, the life force coming through Keith's crown chakra may be stunted and minimal. *Disbeliefs* may also reside in the crown chakra. If a person does not believe in anything greater than herself and refuses to realize the interconnectedness of the life force within, she may experience a block in her crown chakra. This person may feel that she cannot trust others and that she has difficulty protecting herself; she feels alone. Nervous system disorders such as the panic attacks in Keith's case can result. The healing occurs when these individuals can do their own searching and find their own path of Divinity.

THE CROWN CHAKRA: SPIRITUALITY

UNHEALTHY CROWN CHAKRA INDICATIONS

Keith and Keith's mother portrayed dysfunctional crown chakras. See whether you have some healing required in your crown chakra by the number of "Yes" responses to the following questions:

- Do you find that you often obsess about thoughts of God, the afterlife, or spiritual beings?
- Have you isolated yourself from others around you in order to devote your life to something greater than yourself, that is, a higher self or Higher Power?
- Do you tend to have very strong religious or spiritual viewpoints?
- Do you believe that your Divine following is the only way to "get to God"?
- Do you tend to get in debates about your belief systems, always feeling like you have to defend what you believe and make it known to others?
- Do you believe that your earthly existence is an overwhelming bother?
- Do you tend to neglect your earthly needs?
- Do you sometimes feel like you mechanically go through life without any regard for your physical body?
- Do you frequently converse with angels, spirits, or ghosts more than you converse with human beings?
- Do you often feel removed from your physical body?
- Do you often forget to eat?
- Do you lack faith in anything higher or greater than yourself?
- Have you adopted specific beliefs without true introspection and determination of whether they fit your highest self and purpose?
- Do faith-driven people tend to irritate or annoy you?
- When it comes to religious or spiritual beliefs, do you feel confused?
- Do you feel you've been deeply let down by God or a Higher Power?
- Do you neglect to live by your spiritual truths?
- Do you avoid an intimate connection with the Divine due to fear that it could change your life?
- Do you often struggle to maintain your faith in something greater than yourself?

- Do you find that no matter how much you are able to fulfill your material needs, you feel that something deeper or more profound is lacking?

HEALTHY CROWN CHAKRA BEHAVIOR

The crown chakra, residing at the top of the head and extending slightly above the head about 2 inches, truly stands apart from the other six major chakras. From the heart chakra upward begins a successive increase in the proportion of spiritual elements, starting with the heart chakra, which embodies universal love and Christ consciousness; followed by the throat chakra, which symbolizes our own will together with Divine will; and then the third eye chakra, which brings forth the voice of the Divine through our thoughts and consciousness. The crown chakra is more spirit than it is body, and it is our immediate entry point or gateway with Spirit, the Divine, creative, universal life force.

During higher meditation practices or prayer, this center is opened and serves as a conduit to the flow of universal energy and peace. The crown chakra is less about physical embodiment than the other chakras, and it vibrates at the highest rate. Although it is affected by the other chakras, it more often influences them, particularly the root, solar plexus, and throat chakras. The root and the crown chakras share similarities in that the root chakra extracts energy from the Earth for its invigoration, and the crown chakra is nourished by the life force of All That Is. Both the root and crown chakras meet in the middle, at the level of the solar plexus and heart chakras.

This chakra provides us with access to Spirit as needed. It is the entryway for universal light and awareness to penetrate our spirit and earth being. This center harbors much of our beliefs about something greater than us, whether that is religious or spiritual. It acts as a magnet for incoming beliefs about faith and the afterlife. Devoted, spiritual people have a very developed seventh chakra. Like the root chakra that supplies the lower chakras with earth energy, it is important that this center is open so that it can enable the flow of life energy down through to the upper chakras.

The crown chakra is different from the third eye chakra in that the crown chakra is much more directed at the Divine and even higher states of consciousness compared with the third eye chakra, which is much less focused and much more layered with altered dimensions and realities. The crown chakra is the singular highway to the Divine and is completely nonbody. It is the pure essence that we are created from.

A healthy functioning crown chakra will manifest as the ability for individuals to be confident in their faith in a Higher Power, higher self, or in a force that is highly intelligent and creative. Usually, this person will appear as a devout religious or spiritual person who is truly committed to his faith and allows God to guide all decisions in his life. This person may also appear as someone who has strong overarching spiritual principles by which she lives her life. These principles would be founded in a belief in a Higher Power. Examples of people who lived this message would be Mother Teresa and Gandhi.

The third eye chakra is associated with meditation, while the crown chakra connects with prayer—prayer to a being or a force greater than oneself. Prayer may take numerous forms, including devotional chanting (known in the Hindu tradition as *kirtan*), religious hymns, organized, formal prayer, or even words directed to spirit that are created impromptu. All of these forms of devotion have power and potential to connect with the Creator. There are many published studies on the healing nature of prayer. It has been demonstrated that prayer is effective regardless of the faith and regardless of whether the person knows they are being prayed for. The magnitude of these prayers is exponential when more than one person is engaged.

RELIGION VERSUS SPIRITUALITY

The belief in God, or in a force that is greater than us, can be expressed in a variety of ways through the chakras. In the root chakra, these beliefs manifest as a "religion" or an institution, usually composed of a doctrine, rituals, rules, and a community experience. This system binds a tribe together for the benefit of them all by giving them a definite boundary and identity. It is not always acceptable to cross the boundary lines set within a religion. Caroline Myss, in *Anatomy of the Spirit,* eloquently describes religion as "a group experience meant to protect the whole, primarily against physical threats: disease, poverty, death, physical crises, and even war."

As we work our way up the chakras, a belief in a singular godhead becomes a belief in the God in all things. The definition of God expands into an elastic version of religion known as "spirituality." Spirituality recognizes the interconnectedness of life. It may not adhere to any particular text or practices. It could simply be rolled into the way in which we live life—smiling to a stranger on the street, sharing our lunch with a friend, calling our Aunt Lillian just to say hello. Spirituality is a call to emphasize our relationship with Spirit and weave it into our life as Divine threads.

THE BALANCE BETWEEN THE ROOT AND CROWN CHAKRAS

It may seem that the root and crown chakras are polarized in that the root chakra maintains your earthly real estate, and the crown chakra connects you to your spiritual source. Indeed, they are like poles of our energetic fabric, with the root chakra focusing south into the thick of the earth consciousness and the crown chakra going north into the ethers. As Pierre Teilhard de Chardin so famously said, "We are not human beings having a spiritual experience. We are spiritual beings having a human experience." These two chakras encompass the essence of who we are, body and spirit. One of them is not more important than the other. In fact, the best approach is to integrate them as fully as you can by equal attention to your earthly body needs and cultivation of your relationship with a Higher Power. We can merge these energies together in our heart chakra and have it flow through as love. Love has the amazing potential to heal us and others.

Core Issues Associated with the Crown Chakra

- Being able to trust one's higher self
- Believing that there is a power or force greater than oneself
- Knowing that one is supported in all actions by a greater power
- Surrendering one's life to the purpose it was created for

THE NATURE OF THE PURIFICATION VIBRATION

Readings of the crown chakra may reveal a multitude of colors, usually pastels. It may be very bright within the center in an individual who is highly accepting of the Divine, or it may be dark and clouded in an person who lacks trust and faith in any force outside himself. There may be barriers to this opening that appear as metal, hinged plates, or thorns. The extent of the barrier may represent limiting beliefs held by the individual about his or her spiritual views. Many spiritual beings, such as Buddha, Christ, guardian angels, saints, avatars, and spirit guides reside within the crown chakra. They may be part of the crown chakra's energy at birth, or if not from birth, then these beings may appear within the energy of the crown chakra to provide the individual with guidance and support during tender times throughout life.

PHYSIOLOGY AND THE CROWN CHAKRA

The crown chakra is the seat of universal consciousness and potential. It has limited roots in the physical body other than its role of permeating each cell with consciousness. The crown chakra (highest chakra) works together with the root chakra (lowest chakra) to create a harmonized flux of energy throughout the body: the root chakra supplies the physical matter of DNA and cellular organelles, and a ground substance giving them a foundation, whereas the crown chakra is the force that infuses and brings the cells alive, allowing the entire individual to function as a divine creature, intelligent and connected to Spirit. Essentially, the crown chakra animates us.

Aside from the smooth flow of *chi* or *prana* through the circuits of the body that connects it to its soul layer, the crown chakra oversees the workings and electrical activity of the central nervous system throughout the body. The nervous system branches and bundles align closely with the documented channels of energy that course through our body. As mentioned in chapter 2, in traditional Chinese medicine, these networks are known as "energy meridians." Acupuncture is a modality that unifies the chakras by finding blocks in the meridian superhighway overseen by the crown chakra.

> The root chakra maintains your earthly real estate, and the crown chakra connects you to your spiritual source.

THE RELATIONSHIP OF PURIFICATION AND CLARIFICATION TO THE CROWN CHAKRA

CROWN CHAKRA FOOD AND EATING HEALING PLAN

Eat as a Spiritual Practice

The highest expression of the crown chakra as it relates to foods and eating is to turn the entire experience into a means of "in-lightenment" or a spiritual practice. Through our intention to bask in the light of the crown chakra, we infuse sacredness into every moment of the eating event, and, in return, we reap the energy of its miracle. Theology professor Kelton Cobb captured this idea best in the following quote:

The table, the trough, has God's fingerprints all over it. We participate in a mystery whenever we eat food. Indeed, every meal is sacramental. Through eating, death is resurrected into life. Dead fish, dead figs and dead cornflakes are transformed into the living tissue of our bodies. . . . That is an event I would call sacred—a holy occurrence.

What and how we choose to eat says something about our relationship to the Divine. Do we eat in a hurried manner—do we want a shortcut to a holy experience? Are we stuffing our mouths—are we attempting to fill the emptiness within due to the absence of feeling God's presence? Do we numb and distract ourselves with foods rather than look at the deeper, soul-full issues in our lives? Eating is a window into our life with God, and it can also become a conduit for the soul's growth and expression.

Another way to look at our relationship to Spirit is to ask ourselves whether we feel interconnected to all life. As enlightened poet Walt Whitman professed in his verses:

I celebrate myself and sing myself/And what I assume you shall assume/ For every atom belonging to me, as good belongs to you.

The mission of the crown chakra is to ensure that we feel and know that we are part of the web of creation. When this relationship is realized, our crown chakra opens up like the sun rising on the horizon. Our soul is electrified with Spirit's presence.

Include Prayer at Meals

The heart chakra likes to bathe itself in gratitude. Gratitude for eating helps us to center ourselves in the respect for the eating process and all that is involved, from beginning to end. Prayer further anchors our heartfelt gratitude in Divinity. In addition to thanking the plants and animals for giving their lives and the people who helped in the preparation, prayer takes all of these messages and offers them to the whole and to that which is greater than us.

Praying over food ensures that it is blanketed in Divinity and bliss.

When we pray on a meal or for a meal, we recognize the Divinity in the entire offering, and our message of thanks is sent to Spirit. Praying over food ensures that it is blanketed in Divinity and bliss. Prayer protects and transforms our meal into one of sacredness. A spiritual mentor of mine once commented, "Prayer is us talking to God. Intuition is God talking to us." Indeed, when we open up the channel of communication between ourselves and God by engaging the throat and crown chakras, we will receive inspired messages back through the channel of our third eye chakra.

Besides spoken word, prayer may take the form of an action. A beautiful way to acknowledge food as a gift from the Divine is to create a "Spirit plate." The Shamanic tradition has created the practice of asking the animal or plant whether or not it would like to be shared and then offering thanks to that organism. Within this tradition, at the start of a meal, small amounts of foods are placed on a plate and offered as gratitude and sharing to Spirit. The Spirit plate sits on the table during the course of a meal as a reminder of the grace of God. (At the end of the meal it is discarded.)

Release Attachment to Food

When we operate in fear mode, we can become fixated on survival and "having enough." Linda describes how she never felt at peace unless she had a stocked pantry. Her root chakra struggled with issues of abundance. When we come from this place of lack, we eat out of the need to "be filled" rather than finding the source of fulfillment through God and trusting that we will have enough if we rely on the strength of our crown chakra to guide us. The lesson of this chakra is that real nourishment comes not from food but from our spirituality—our connection to God. It contains a knowing that transcends earthly tools and information and rests in a realm of utter peace, trust, and abundance.

"Prayer is us talking to God. Intuition is God talking to us."

Purify the Body through Fasting

As stated earlier, the crown chakra is the least physical chakra; it is more spirit than physical flesh. It holds space for our soul. Since it is not physical, it does not require food. It feeds off of spiritual morsels of prayer and Divine inspiration. Our physical and spiritual bodies are merged. So, when we fast, we cast off the physical energy and residue that prevent us from having a clean, clear spirit. We replace the physical nourishment with spiritual sustenance.

Most religious and spiritual traditions include either a time of the year or an ongoing discipline when certain foods are omitted from or included in the diet. The Islamic tradition of Ramadan is a forty-day-long fast when no food is eaten until sundown. Similarly, the Roman Catholic period of Lent includes eating fish on Fridays. It is a common practice during Lent to give up some item or practice, and often this omission is a food.

Releasing ourselves in some degree from the practice of eating may allow the body's needs to be temporarily suspended so that the needs of the spirit may be tended to. Of course, due to health reasons, some individuals may not be able to do a fast. Others may want to do a fast under the supervision of a trained medical professional. There are many manifestations of fasting. A fast may be as simple as skipping lunch on Sundays, or it may be several days of replacing all solid food with fresh-squeezed juices (not advised under certain health conditions).

Fasting may provide clarity on some spiritual issues. The classical example might be the story of Jesus, who fasted for forty days and forty nights in the desert and during that time was faced with his temptations. Fasting may cause us to take a look at who we are beyond our bodies. Again, note that there are varying degrees of fasting and that not everyone's health condition allows them to engage in such a practice.

Bask in Simplicity

Since it is nonphysical, the crown chakra does not need to spend its time with physical activities such as meal selection and preparation. In fact, it vibrates to just the opposite—simplicity. It hums to the sacred simplicity of a piece of fresh fruit, a vegetable picked from the garden, or a glass of pure water. Whole foods in their natural form are most resonant with the crown chakra. Processed foods add in layers of complexity and other energies that can make the crown chakra energy murky.

In addition to eating simple foods, we can eat without much fuss. Don Gerrard has written the book *One Bowl* to introduce the concept of an individual eating every meal from the same bowl. By deliberately focusing our intention on a particular eating vessel, we can concentrate it with healing, loving thoughts and action. Just like the heart chakra, the crown chakra is receptive to this type of practice.

Feast on Pure, Unadulterated Foods

Like fasting, foods that are pure keep the metabolic machinery of the physical body flowing and integrated with the spirit. Pure foods include plants that are grown in the absence of pesticides, herbicides, insecticides, with their DNA intact (not genetically modified). Heirloom seeds and plants are great for this purpose. For animal foods to be considered pure, they would need to be fed high-quality non-GMO feed, be free to range, and not be injected with unnecessary hormones or antibiotics. It is ideal to have these plants and animals cultivated in a loving environment, in accordance with natural principles.

In contrast, a number of artificial, synthetic foods—such as artificial sweeteners, soft drinks, partially hydrogenated (trans) fats, and GMO foods—are damaging to the qualities of the crown chakra.

SUBSTANCES FOR PURIFICATION AND CLARIFICATION

The radiant sun symbolizes foods for the crown chakra. In a multitude of ways, the sun gives us sustenance. It helps plants to photosynthesize, it gives us the energy of warmth, it sets the course for our biological rhythms. The sun spans its rays like the crown chakra extends its unifying energy to our highest self. The vibrant beams of the crown chakra radiate through all the chakras, unifying them. The symbol of the sun speaks to the essence of the crown chakra, which is not about the physical gift of food but the nourishment we receive from the nonphysicals: sunlight, air, and love.

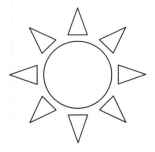

Sunlight

The crown chakra has often been referred to as the sun, or as being gold in color. Like the individual photons vibrating within the glorious sun rays, the magnificent crown chakra resonates to the fine vibration of the source of universal light. Sunlight and crown chakra energy can permeate our physical being and spark certain cell processes. Ultraviolet light has been shown to activate a vitamin D precursor in our skin to its active form. Vitamin D supports the crown chakra function. In a world where we lived only from our crown chakra, we might be able to live on sunshine alone.

Air

Oxygen, extracted from breath (referred to as *chi* or *prana*), is the subtle substance that keeps the cells of an individual vibrant and flowing. Simply put, an organism would not survive without it. Oxygen is the key component that the body uses to access the energy contained within bonds of glucose in a process called oxidative metabolism (also called cellular respiration). We cannot assimilate the vibration of foods to feed our chakras unless we have the essential wiring in place to our crown chakra. With oxygen, our being stays conscious, alive, and invigorated. Deep breathing and oxygenation therapies help to clear the crown chakra.

Certain incense and smudging herbs can be purifying for the crown chakra. Herbs such as dried white sage, copal, myrrh, frankincense, and juniper are not meant to be eaten but are ritually burned in a safe container; the light smoke fills the room, and we inhale through the nostrils. Some of these herbs can be smoked through a ceremonial pipe for purification purposes.

Detoxification

Numerous books have been written on detoxification practices. Each person is varied in his or her detoxification needs. Over time, it is natural to get a build-up of toxic products in our bodies from the air we breathe and from the foods we eat. Every season, it is a nourishing practice to undergo a detoxification of our external and internal environment to purify the body and clarify the mind. When we detoxify, it is like pushing an internal reset button. Once again, we can think straight, our eyes are clear, our skin is glowing.

There are many ways to do a detoxification. Some people like juicing, others a water fast, and there is a detoxification process that involves nutritional support like vitamins and minerals. Using nutritional support may be optimal, as supplementation can provide us with necessary nutrients to assist in the disposal of what we no longer need. Physical detoxification can be complemented with emotional, mental, and spiritual detoxification. During detoxification, the focus is on "What do you need to let go of?" This could be old emotional patterns, thoughts, and beliefs.

To ensure the thoroughness of our purification cycle, we may want to connect the crown chakra to other chakras for release of energy in these centers (see Table 10.1). For example, one could start with purification of the root chakra by releasing old ancestral patterns and by encouraging the elimination process. From there, the sacral chakra could be cleansed using the element of water by drinking fasts, sweating, and hydrotherapy (heated baths containing mineral salts). The solar plexus chakra could purge its extra fire through the movement of exercise and the release of disempowering thoughts and actions. The heart chakra could be cleansed through sound and deep breathing to expel toxins in the chest. As discussed earlier, the throat chakra is the hub of communication. What toxic language are we communicating that needs disposal? The third eye chakra can be cleared through good-quality sleep and rest. By encouraging mental rest, we allow toxic thoughts to settle so they can be swept away. And finally, the crown chakra could pull together its fragmented, disconnected energy into an energy of wholeness through deep breathing and soaking in the sun rays through skin or sight.

We could also transition to a more rigorous detoxification program by eating "light" or in smaller portions. Caloric restriction in animals has been shown to result in the animals' life span increasing. Thus, by reducing our energy input through physical matter, we create more room for our spiritual substance to permeate our flesh. Fewer toxins are formed, and we are rewarded with a longer life.

Love

In the end, there is nothing that we can feel more nourished by than love. It is different than food in that the more we allow it to feed us, the more it grows, enabling others to be fed. When we are ready to accept love fully and completely, without limits, we will be liberated from having to ingest any food to feed our vibration. If we are in a body, chances are that we are just not at that point. We may be in a body to learn and grow through the very lesson of love on this planet. We have the chakras to guide us to reaching our love potential.

Table 10.1   Chakra Detoxification

Week	Chakra	Modalities	Release/Replace
I	Root	Increased fiber	Release fear and outdated ancestral patterns that no longer serve you, replace with safety and trust
2	Sacral	Increased water intake, sweating through sauna (especially steam sauna), use of salt baths	Release blocks in creative flow and emotions, replace with embraced personal expression
3	Solar plexus	Movement of any type, dry sauna, full-body massage	Release unnecessary control, disempowered thoughts, and frustration, replace with courage and personal power
4	Heart	Listening to music, singing, deep breathing	Release hatred and bitterness, replace with compassion and love
5	Throat	Examine and extract toxic language in our speech	Release deception and artificiality, replace with truth and authenticity
6	Third eye	Nourishing sleep, dream analysis	Release overthinking and illusion, replace with detachment and intuition
7	Crown	Deep breathing, sunlight	Release fragmentation and separation, replace with unification and purpose

AFFIRMATIONS TO HEAL THE CROWN CHAKRA

Affirmations are helpful tools that assist us in changing core belief patterns. By writing these words or by saying them on a daily basis, we infuse our subconscious with new patterns. As we continue to make them a part of our surroundings, so will they become part of who we are. Make up your own as you see appropriate. Here are some to get you started.

* *When I eat, I connect with Spirit.*
* *I "in-lighten" my soul with the sacred practice of eating.*
* *I release my body of toxins.*
* *Love and light fill me, and I am complete.*

- *I invite the radiance of my soul to penetrate every cell of my being.*
- *I fill myself with the delight and mystery of the cosmos.*

FOOD AND EATING ACTIVITIES
TO BALANCE THE CROWN CHAKRA

- Before eating, try "bathing" your food in sunlight. Allow your plateful of food to bask in the sun for a couple of minutes, allowing it to be invigorated with the high photonic energy of Divine radiance.
- Create a prayer to say before eating.
- Make a food offering to the Divine in the form of a Spirit plate.
- How do you eat? What does this suggest about your relationship with God?
- Create or buy a bowl that you use for all meals. Try using it exclusively for one week. Journal on your experience.
- Instead of a "mind-full" exercise with food, try a "Spirit-full" experience with food. With each bite, imagine unlocking the spirituality that pervades the matrix of the food. How does this connection help to put you into touch with God?
- Do a detoxification program that you create based on the needs of your body and soul.
- List ten ways that you can invite more love into your daily life.

EATING PLAN TO SUPPORT PURIFICATION

Sipping in clean air
Eating in the sunlight
Drinking pure water
Sun-and-Fruit Water*
Clean, organic foods of highest quality
Fresh juices and broths to support detoxification
Detox Dynamo*
Berry Flush*
Green Goddess*
Divine Broth*

---

* Indicates recipe at back of book

And when you crush an apple with your teeth,
say to it in your heart,
"Your seeds shall live in my body,
And the buds of your tomorrow shall blossom in my heart,
And your fragrance shall be my breath,
And together we shall rejoice through all the seasons."
—KAHLIL GIBRAN, *Eating and Drinking*, CHAPTER VI

FREQUENTLY ASKED QUESTIONS

Making the beginning is one third of the work.
—IRISH PROVERB

If I crave a food, does this mean my chakras are unbalanced?

The easiest way to think about food is as a metaphor or a symbol. If you are craving a food, what are you craving more of in your life? The energy of cravings, or the desire to consume specific foods, is held within the sacral chakra. If the apparent meaning of the craving doesn't simply jump out at you, take a look at your sacral chakra. Are you expressing emotions, creating, and having fun? Sacral chakra imbalance may be putting you on craving overdrive.

What is the easiest way to begin eating in sync with my chakras?

It is as easy as answering the questions at the beginning of each chapter describing the chakras. Is there a chakra that is calling your attention? If so, start there. Check your chakra status as you are experiencing significant emotional, physical, mental, or spiritual changes.

Can I balance my chakras through foods and eating alone?

There are many ways to help align your energy centers, and no one of them truly works effectively on its own. Aligning foods and eating with the needs of the chakras present one powerful way to begin and support a shift in your consciousness since eating occurs every day, many times a day. Eating certain foods will assist in shifting your chakras, giving you a new "baseline" that is better equipped to hold changes you are trying to implement in your life.

Altering eating patterns over the long term can have a significant effect on one's life. This effect is magnified and strengthened by coupling it with other activities like adjusting the type and amount of exercise you engage in every day, transforming negative thoughts into those that are positive and self-affirming, tweaking daily tasks, refreshing your career, and even tailoring the color clothes you wear to your chakras.

How fast does my chakra shift after I've eaten a food?

Remember that eating begins before we've taken our first bite. Eating is the whole process and experience around food. Thus, our chakras are engaged throughout the day. Just looking at a food and taking in the color and form can spark alchemy in the chakras. When we eat a food, the chakras are set into full motion. Imagine the wheels of the chakras as always spinning; they can alter their speed, openness, or vibration with any interaction with food.

How is this book different from "diet" books?

Reading a book is a two-way street. How much do you interact with and invest yourself into the information? How much did you know about the subject matter before you started reading? What are your judgments, biases? If you are drawn to read a book, there may be good reason. For example, you may uncover the one shining nugget that illuminates your path and changes your life radically.

Use this book as a tool to help you enter your chakra world and to understand how to connect all aspects of yourself through the healing properties of food and eating. This book has built a bridge between our energy centers and food to help you merge the physical and spiritual aspects of yourself. It is a key to understanding how to use your body's wisdom within the realm of food choices and eating practices.

I struggle with my weight—why is this?

There is no single-bullet answer to this complex question. Explore your inner depths through your chakras to mine the root of this issue. The root, sacral, and solar plexus chakras are often at play in overweight individuals. See if there is some healing required in these centers, using food and other modalities.

What happens if I eat "unhealthy" foods? Will I damage my chakras?

Two questions spring to mind when I hear this type of question: (1) What do you consider "unhealthy"? and (2) Why are you making the choice (think throat chakra!) to eat these foods? Most of us eat a variety of foods throughout the day. Are all of them truly unhealthy, and "unhealthy" according to whom? This term is relative and implies judgment (solar plexus chakra). It puts us into a mode of analysis-paralysis. On the other hand, if you put yourself in situations that have you gravitating to "unhealthy" foods, see if you can understand why.

To compensate, try to ensure that your style of eating is nourishing—that is, that you pray or give gratitude before eating and that you eat in a medium to slow, conscious manner. Infuse the food with love as much as possible. Do a three-second visualization with the food, imagining that every cell of the food is dancing to the tune of love.

How often do I have to eat certain foods for my chakras to benefit?
The frequency of eating particular foods that resonate to a particular chakra is dependent on your body and chakra wisdom. Ask your root chakra to assist you with eating more instinctually and your third eye chakra to unfold to you a more intuitive rhythm of food selection.

RECIPES FOR THE CHAKRAS

■ ■ ■ ■ ■ ■ ■ ■ ■

*Cooking is like love. It should be entered into
with abandon or not at all.*
—HARRIET VAN HORNE

TO SUPPORT THE ROOT CHAKRA

CINNAMON-NUT BAKED APPLE

The mighty apple to treat your core
Serves 2

2 Tbsp. cashew pieces
2 Tbsp. pecan pieces
1 Tbsp. unsweetened coconut flakes
1 tsp. cinnamon
2 Tbsp. agave nectar or honey
2 apples, cored
2 Tbsp. apple juice concentrate
1 cup water
2 Tbsp. nonfat, plain yogurt (optional)

In a small bowl, mix together the nut pieces, unsweetened coconut flakes, cinnamon, and agave nectar. Place cored apples in a small glass baking dish. Spoon mixture into the center of each apple and any remainder over the tops of the apples. Combine apple juice concentrate and water and pour over apples. Bake uncovered at 350°F for 30 minutes or until apples become soft. Serve with a dollop of nonfat yogurt as topping.

STIR-FRIED GINGER-GARLIC TOFU WITH VEGETABLES

The power of ancient roots and plant protein to nourish you from within
Serves 4

1 pound extra firm tofu
2 Tbsp. tamari (low-sodium soy sauce)
2 Tbsp. sesame oil
2 tsp. peeled and minced fresh ginger
2 minced garlic cloves
2 cups broccoli florets
2 cups sliced mushrooms
1 red bell pepper cut into thin strips
Salt and pepper to taste

Drain and cube tofu. Toss with tamari soy sauce and 1 Tbsp. oil in a small bowl and set aside for 5–10 minutes. In a wok or large nonstick skillet, heat 1 Tbsp. oil over high heat and add ginger and garlic; stir-fry for 30 seconds. Add marinated tofu, stir-frying for 2 more minutes. Toss in broccoli, mushrooms, and bell pepper, and continue stir-frying for 2 minutes. Salt and pepper can be added for taste.

EARTHY CHILI

Connects you to the core of Earth energy
Serves 8

2 Tbsp. olive oil
1 medium onion, chopped
4 cloves garlic, minced
$^1/_2$ pound mushrooms, chopped
2 15-oz. cans pinto or kidney beans, including liquid
1 red bell pepper, chopped
2 cups cauliflower pieces
2 carrots, scrubbed and chopped
1 28-oz. can plum tomatoes, with juice

2 Tbsp. tomato paste
3 Tbsp. red wine vinegar or red wine
1 cup tomato juice
1 Tbsp. ground cumin
2 Tbsp. chili powder
1 tsp. paprika
Salt and pepper to taste

In large soup pan, over medium heat, sauté onions and garlic in the olive oil until onions become yellow and soft, about 5 minutes. Add mushrooms, and sauté another 5–10 minutes. Stir in remaining ingredients and bring mixture to a boil. Reduce heat to simmer. Cover and cook, stirring occasionally, until vegetables are tender, about 50 minutes. Serve hot.

NOURISHING BEAN SOUP

Excellent soup for feeling more centered during times of stress
Serves 6

2 cups white kidney beans (cannellini)
1–2 cups kidney, adzuki, or red beans (canned or cooked from dry)
1 cup chickpeas (garbanzos canned or cooked from dry)
2–3 cups fresh spinach or escarole, washed, drained and chopped, *or* 1
    10-oz. package frozen chopped spinach
4 cups chicken or vegetable broth
2 onions, chopped
2 cloves garlic, minced
1 tsp. each dried basil and oregano
1 Tbsp. dried parsley
Pepper to taste

Combine all ingredients and simmer for 45 minutes. Serve hot.

TURKEY LOAF

Don't forget to give thanks to the turkey!
Serves 4–6

1 pound ground free-range turkey
1 egg, beaten
$^1/_2$ cup crimini mushrooms, sautéed in butter
$^1/_2$ cup water
$^1/_2$ cup celery, chopped
1 small cooked red potato, diced
$^1/_4$ cup organic oats
$^1/_4$ cup almond meal
1 Tbsp. dried parsley
2 tsp. dried tarragon
1 tsp. dried sage
Sea salt and fresh ground pepper to taste

Preheat oven to 375°F. Mix all ingredients together in a bowl. Put into a casserole dish. Bake for 35–40 minutes.

CREAMY COLD TOMATO SOUP

Refreshing groundedness! Great for connecting and clearing the throat and root chakras . . .
Serves 5

1 cucumber, chopped
1 scallion, chopped
1 clove garlic
4 cups tomato juice, unsalted
1 red or green pepper, chopped
$^1/_2$ tsp. oregano
1 cup plain yogurt
Sliced mushrooms or tomato chunks for garnish
Salt and pepper

Combine all ingredients (except yogurt) in small amounts in blender and blend until smooth. Whisk in yogurt. Chill several hours before serving and garnish as desired with mushrooms or tomato. Add salt and pepper to taste.

WINTER ROOT VEGETABLE SOUP

Very grounding combination of root vegetables to set your feet firmly on the Earth
Serves 4

2 Tbsp. olive oil
1-$^1/_2$ cups coarsely chopped onions
3 Tbsp. finely chopped garlic
6 cups chicken stock
2 Tbsp. apple-cider vinegar
1 pound celery root, diced (about 2-$^1/_2$ cups)
$^3/_4$ pound red potatoes, diced (about 2-$^1/_3$ cups)
$^3/_4$ pound sweet potatoes, diced (about 2-$^1/_3$ cups)
$^1/_2$ pound parsnips, diced (1-$^3/_4$ cups)
$^1/_2$ pound carrots, diced (1-$^1/_3$ cups)
$^1/_4$ pound turnips, diced (2 cups)
$^1/_2$ tsp. minced fresh gingerroot
$^1/_2$ tsp. salt
$^1/_4$ tsp. cumin
$^1/_4$ tsp. curry
$^1/_8$ tsp. cayenne pepper

Heat the oil in a saucepan over high heat. Add the onions and sauté until soft and yellow. Add the garlic and sauté 1 minute. Add to a large soup pot along with the remaining ingredients. Simmer for 90 minutes. Serve hot.

RED WHIRL SMOOTHIE

A great grounding energizer to start your day!
Serves 4

2 cups frozen strawberries
1 cup frozen raspberries
8 oz. plain, unsweetened yogurt
1 cup milk (soy milk or cow's milk)
2 Tbsp. agave nectar
1 Tbsp. bee pollen (optional)
Handful of ice cubes

Combine ingredients in a blender; fill to the top with ice cubes. Blend until smooth.

MORNING SCRAMBLE

Excellent for balancing root and heart chakras!
Serves 2

3 medium-sized red potatoes, washed and cubed into 8 sections
2 Tbsp. olive oil
2 cloves garlic, minced
1 green onion
$^1/_8$ cup black olives, sliced
1 cup broccoli florets
4 eggs
2 Tbsp. milk (soymilk or cow's milk)
2 Tbsp. feta cheese
Pinch curry powder
Salt and pepper

Boil red potatoes in a skillet until they are slightly soft but not mushy. Pour off any excess water from the skillet and add olive oil. Stir-fry potatoes together with garlic, green onion, olives, and broccoli florets on low heat for 2 minutes. In a small bowl, whisk together eggs, milk, 1 Tbsp. feta cheese, and curry. Pour egg mixture over stir-fry and heat, using spatula to combine ingredients periodically. Add salt and pepper to taste. Sprinkle 1 Tbsp. crumbled feta on top.

TO SUPPORT THE SACRAL CHAKRA

HONEYED PAPAYA WITH RAW COCONUT FLAKES

Allow the healing vibration of the tropics to infuse your creative spirit!
Serves 1 or 2

1 ripe papaya
1 tsp. honey
$^1/_2$ cup raw coconut flakes

Slice papaya in half, clean out seeds. Drizzle 1 tsp. honey over both halves. Sprinkle with raw coconut flakes and serve immediately.

PLEASURE FRUIT MIX

Let this mixture provide you with a blend of pleasure, play, and passion!
Serves 4

2 peaches, sliced
2 ripe bananas, diced
1 nectarine, sliced
1 blood orange, sectioned
1 mango, cut into thin slices
$^1/_2$ cup unsweetened shredded coconut
2 Tbsp. lime or lemon juice
Mint sprig (optional)

Mix all ingredients except for lime or lemon juice in a large bowl. Drizzle lime or lemon juice over entire mixture. Cover and refrigerate or serve immediately. Place mint sprig on top.

FLOWING GINGER-MANGO SMOOTHIE

A morning creativity booster!
Serves 2

1 ripe mango, peeled and sliced
1 can of light coconut milk
2 Tbsp. ground flaxseed meal
Pinch ground ginger

Blend all ingredients in blender until smooth. Serve immediately or freeze
for 1 hour to serve as a sorbet.

GRILLED SALMON WITH APRICOT ORANGE SAUCE
AND BABY CARROTS

A meal packed with sacral chakra goodness all the way through . . .
Serves 4

24 ounces wild salmon

Sauce:
$^3/_4$ cup apricot preserves
1 Tbsp. teriyaki sauce
2 Tbsp. balsamic vinegar
$^1/_2$ tsp. ginger, finely chopped
2 Tbsp. sesame oil
2 Tbsp. orange juice
1 tsp. orange zest
1 small bag baby carrots

Cut salmon into four 6-oz. servings and set aside in a 9 × 13-inch baking
pan. In small saucepan, combine apricot preserves, teriyaki sauce, vinegar,
and ginger. Stir over low heat for about a minute or until preserves become
liquid. Set aside to cool to room temperature. Add sesame oil, orange juice,
and orange zest and mix well. Pour $^3/_4$ of mixture on top of salmon. Cover
with tinfoil and refrigerate for 1–2 hours or until ready to grill. Keep remaining sauce on side in a small bowl.

Meanwhile, allow baby carrots to steam until they reach a soft consistency.

Preheat grill to medium. Grease grill. Remove marinated salmon and place on grill. Cover grill and cook 3–4 minutes per side or until desired doneness. Serve salmon with warm apricot sauce and baby carrots.

CREATIVE CARROT CURRY ("3C") SOUP

Allow your creative juices to flow with this delicate combination of carrot and curry
Serves 4

1 Tbsp. olive oil
1 medium yellow onion, chopped finely
2 pounds carrots, scrubbed and unpeeled, cut into $^1/_2$-inch thick rounds
1 Tbsp. curry powder
5 cups vegetable or chicken broth
1 cup light coconut milk
Salt and freshly ground pepper to taste

Heat the olive oil in large saucepan over medium heat. Add the chopped onion and stir 3–4 minutes or until it turns golden. Add carrots and stir well. Stir in curry powder and cook, stirring constantly, for 30 seconds. Add the broth and bring to boil over high heat. Reduce heat to medium-low and partially cover the saucepan. Simmer about 30 minutes, or until carrots are tender. In small increments, transfer soup to a blender or food processor, blending until smooth. Pour the puréed soup into large bowl. Stir in coconut milk over low heat. Season with salt and pepper and serve hot.

WILD RICE-ALMOND STUFFED ORANGE BELL PEPPER

Wonderful to balance all three lower chakras
Serves 2

$^1/_3$ cup chopped yellow onion
1 clove garlic, minced
1 Tbsp. olive oil

2 cups vegetable or chicken broth
1 cup wild rice
$^1/_8$ cup celery, diced
$^1/_8$ cup carrot, sliced into $^1/_2$-inch rounds
$^1/_2$ cup almond slivers
$^1/_8$ tsp. rosemary
$^1/_8$ tsp. oregano
Pinch sea salt
2 large orange bell peppers, stems removed

In large saucepan, sauté onion and garlic in 1 Tbsp. olive oil until onion becomes soft. Add broth, rice, celery, and carrot. Bring to boil; cover, reduce heat, and simmer for 20–25 minutes or until rice is almost done. Remove from heat. Add $^1/_4$ cup almond slivers and spices. Set aside. Place peppers in large saucepan filled with 2 inches water. Bring to boil and cook for 2–3 minutes or until slightly tender. Drain water from saucepan. Place peppers in small glass casserole dish. Stuff with rice-almond mixture and spoon excess around peppers. Cover with foil and bake at 350°F for 15 minutes. Sprinkle top of peppers with remaining almonds and serve.

YAM PECAN BAKE

A tasty, tantalizing treat for your sacral chakra—could also be a dessert!
Serves 4

5 medium-sized yams
1 15-oz. can lite coconut milk
$^1/_4$ cup agave nectar
$^1/_4$ cup pecans, chopped
$^1/_4$ cup unsweetened, shredded coconut
$^1/_2$ tsp. cinnamon
Dash nutmeg

Bake yams in oven for 1 hour at 350°F or until soft. Peel skin off and put yams into large bowl. Break into small pieces using a fork. Pour coconut milk onto yams, stirring and mashing the mixture to make it smooth. Add agave nectar, pecans, shredded coconut and mix well. Pour into medium-sized casserole dish. Sprinkle top with pecans and shredded coconut. Serve either warm or cold.

MACADAMIA NUT—ENCRUSTED HALIBUT

Triple flow potential with healing oils from flaxseed, nuts, and fish
Serves 4

1 cup brown rice flour
$^1/_4$ cup flaxseed meal
3 eggs
$^1/_4$ cup orange juice
2 cups lightly salted roasted macadamia nuts, finely chopped
4 halibut fillets
$^1/_4$ cup clarified butter (ghee), melted
2 Tbsp. finely chopped green onion for garnish

Combine flour and flaxseed meal in a shallow bowl or plate. In a separate shallow mixing bowl, beat eggs and orange juice. Put macadamia nuts on a third shallow bowl or plate. Flour both sides of a fillet, dip in the egg bowl, and then completely cover both sides with nuts. Repeat the same procedure for all fillets. Place the fillets on a heated skillet with melted ghee and fry both sides until fish is cooked, about 10 minutes total. Sprinkle fillet with chopped green onion. Serve with mango chutney on side (see throat chakra recipes).

FRESH ALMOND AND CASHEW NUT BUTTER

Dynamic blend to nourish the root and sacral chakras
About 2 cups

1 cup unsalted roasted shelled almonds
1 cup lightly salted dry roasted cashews
2 Tbsp. organic sunflower or safflower oil
$^1/_4$ tsp. sea salt
$^1/_2$ tsp. cinnamon

Blend all the ingredients together in a heavy-duty blender or food processor. Store in the refrigerator in an airtight glass jar. Use within 2 weeks.

WALNUT PESTO

Great as an addition to whole grain crackers or vegetables; strengthens the sacral and heart chakras

3 cups

1 large head elephant garlic
1 cup olive oil
$^1/_2$ cup fresh basil leaves
1 cup walnuts (shelled)
$^1/_2$ cup black walnuts
1 cup pine nuts
$^1/_8$ cup walnut oil

Bake garlic in covered oiled glass dish in oven at 350°F for about 40 minutes. Baste occasionally with olive oil. Cool and peel. Chop the basil leaves and add to blender or food processor. Add garlic, nuts, and remaining oil and mix well. Cover mixture with thin layer of walnut oil and keep in refrigerator for up to 2 weeks.

TO SUPPORT THE SOLAR PLEXUS CHAKRA

FIERY CURRY LENTIL SOUP

Gives incredible staying power—perfect for aligning chakras 1 through 6
Serves 6

4 large garlic cloves, peeled and finely chopped
2 medium yellow onions, finely diced
1 Tbsp. expeller-pressed olive oil
2 cups brown and/or yellow lentils
1 cup of fresh corn pieces
3–4 carrots, sliced
3 large yellow potatoes, cut into 1-inch cubes
$^1/_4$ tsp. cumin
2 tsp. curry
Dash sea salt
10 cups of vegetable or chicken broth

In a small saucepan, heat garlic and onions in olive oil over medium heat until soft. Wash lentils thoroughly. In a large stock pot, add broth and all other ingredients, including the sautéed garlic and onions. Simmer and stir occasionally for at least one hour. Serve warm. Freeze unused portions.

BROWN RICE PUDDING

A transformative treat!
Serves 4

2 cups brown rice
4 cups water
$^1/_2$ cup coconut milk
1 tsp. cinnamon
$^1/_2$ tsp. cardamom
1 scant handful pecan pieces
$^1/_4$ cup agave nectar

Rinse rice well. Add to medium saucepan with 4 cups water. Cover and cook 20–25 minutes or until rice is done. To cooked rice, stir in coconut milk, cinnamon, cardamom, and pecan pieces. Stir in agave nectar. Serve warm or cold.

POWER BROWN RICE WITH YELLOW VEGETABLES AND SESAME-TAMARI DRESSING

A food fusion for solar plexus and sacral chakras
Serves 4

1 cup whole grain (short or long grain) organic brown rice (for a nuttier texture, choose short grain)
2 Tbsp. sesame seeds, toasted
3 Tbsp. rice vinegar
2 Tbsp. tamari sauce
1 Tbsp. toasted sesame oil
4 tsp. minced fresh ginger
2 garlic cloves, minced or pressed

2 tsp. agave nectar
1 cup cubed yellow squash
1 cup diced yellow bell pepper
$^1/_2$ cup chopped green onions

Combine rice with 2-$^1/_2$ cups of water in medium saucepan. Bring to a simmer over medium-high heat. Reduce heat to low and simmer, covered, until rice is tender and water has been absorbed, 30–35 minutes. Fluff with fork and transfer to large bowl. Alternately, cook rice in rice cooker.

While rice is cooking, toast sesame seeds in small dry skillet over medium-low heat, stirring constantly until golden and fragrant, about 3 minutes. Cool in small bowl. Whisk together vinegar, tamari sauce, oil, ginger, garlic, and agave nectar in another small bowl. Add this mixture to rice when cooled and toss to coat well. Add yellow squash, yellow bell pepper, and green onion, and toss to coat. Sprinkle with sesame seeds before serving.

QUINOA-AMARANTH PINE NUT SALAD

A sustaining staple!
Serves 2

1 cup quinoa, rinsed
1 cup amaranth, rinsed
3 cups water
Pinch sea salt
$^1/_2$ cup corn kernels
$^1/_2$ medium cucumber, diced
1 medium tomato, diced
$^1/_2$ cup chopped cilantro
$^1/_2$ cup chopped basil
2 Tbsp. lemon juice
1 cup pine nuts
Pepper

Combine quinoa, amaranth, water, and salt in a medium-sized covered saucepan. Bring to boil, simmer 20 minutes. In medium-sized glass bowl, mix together corn, cucumber, tomato, cilantro, basil, and lemon juice. Add to quinoa mixture. Mix well. Toss in pine nuts before serving. Sprinkle with pepper to taste. Serve warm or cold.

MIXED MUESLI

An excellent cereal for integrating lower chakras: solar plexus, sacral, and root
Serves 2–4

1 cup puffed rice cereal
$^1/_2$ cup crispy brown rice
$^1/_8$ cup wheat bran
$^1/_8$ cup flaxseeds
$^1/_8$ cup unsweetened shredded coconut
$^1/_4$ cup sliced almonds
$^1/_8$ cup chopped pecans
$^1/_8$ cup pumpkin seeds
$^1/_4$ cup raisins
$^1/_4$ cup agave nectar
$^1/_4$ cup clarified butter (ghee), melted

Mix all ingredients together in a large mixing bowl. Spread contents flat on cookie sheet. Bake at 375°F for 20 minutes or until slightly browned. Store at room temperature in a plastic or glass jar. Use as a portable snack or cereal.

MEDITERRANEAN POLENTA MEDALLIONS

Energize your solar plexus with the flavor of the Mediterranean!
Serves 2

1 roll precooked compressed polenta, sliced
2 Tbsp. olive oil
$^1/_2$ cup basil, chopped
1 tsp. oregano
1 medium tomato, diced
$^1/_2$ cup pine nuts

$^1/_4$ cup feta cheese
Dash sea salt
Dash pepper

Arrange polenta slices on an oiled skillet and heat over medium heat, flipping over after about 1 minute or when polenta turns slightly brown. Empty toasted polenta onto large plate. On top of polenta, add basil, oregano, tomato, pine nuts, feta cheese, and salt and pepper to taste.

SUNNY CORN SALAD

Super salad for summer picnics—helps bring out the sunshine in your solar plexus chakra
Serves 2–4

6 to 8 ears fresh corn or 3 cups frozen corn kernels
1 large red bell pepper, diced
3 green onions, cut into $^1/_4$-inch pieces
$^1/_8$ cup olive oil
2 Tbsp. lemon juice
1–2 cloves garlic, minced
$^1/_4$ cup cilantro
$^1/_8$ tsp. chili powder
1–2 jalapenos, diced
Salt and pepper to taste

Combine all ingredients in a medium-sized glass mixing bowl. Serve cold.

TO SUPPORT THE HEART CHAKRA

THE HEART SALAD

A classic, nourishing treat for the heart chakra
Serves 4

1 bag fresh organic spinach leaves (10–12 oz.)
1 ripe avocado, diced into cubes

1 cup broccoli sprouts
1 tsp. fresh dill
$^1/_2$ cup strawberries, sliced in half (to resemble heart shape)
$^1/_2$ cup toasted slivered almonds
Dash sea salt and pepper

Dressing
$^1/_4$ cup organic flaxseed oil
$^1/_4$ cup extra virgin olive oil
$^1/_4$ cup balsamic vinegar

Wash spinach leaves and put into large serving bowl. Add avocado cubes, broccoli sprouts, and dill, and lightly mix throughout. Top with strawberries and almonds. Combine dressing ingredients in shaker cup. When ready to serve, drizzle salad with dressing.

ROSEMARY ROASTED CAULIFLOWER AND PINE NUTS

Allows the love within
Serves 4

1 head organic cauliflower
2 cloves of garlic, peeled and minced
$^1/_8$ cup extra virgin olive oil
1 Tbsp. fresh rosemary
$^1/_2$ cup raw pine nuts
Sea salt
Fresh ground pepper

Preheat oven to 425°F. Break apart cauliflower into bite-sized pieces or florets and place in large mixing bowl. Add garlic and stir throughout. Pour in olive oil and ensure that all cauliflower pieces are drizzled with oil. Sprinkle with rosemary, pine nuts, salt, and pepper. Transfer mixture evenly onto baking sheet and bake, uncovered, in oven for 20–25 minutes or until the top and edges of cauliflower are lightly brown. Serve immediately.

HEART-WARMING BRUSSELS SPROUTS

Deliciously divine and devoted to you
Serves 4

1 pound fresh Brussels sprouts, washed and cut in half
1 small yellow onion, peeled and chopped
2 Tbsp. ghee
Dash sea salt and pepper
2 Tbsp. freshly grated Parmesan cheese

Steam Brussels sprouts for 2–3 minutes or until bright green and tender. Sauté onions in 1 Tbsp. ghee until they become translucent. Add steamed Brussels sprouts and the remaining ghee. Toss, sprinkle with salt and pepper to taste, and cook on medium-high heat until Brussels sprouts turn slightly brown. Remove from heat, put into serving dish. Sprinkle top with grated Parmesan cheese.

FLAX-ZUCCHINI MUFFINS OF JOY

For happiness and gratitude in the mornings
9–10 large muffins

1-$^1/_2$ cups brown rice flour
1 cup flaxseed meal
2 tsp. baking soda
1 tsp. baking powder
$^1/_2$ tsp. sea salt
2 tsp. cinnamon
$^1/_2$ tsp. cardamom
$^1/_2$ cup raisins
1 cup pecans, chopped
1 cup agave nectar
1-$^1/_2$ cups zucchini, shredded
$^3/_4$ cup soy milk
2 eggs, beaten
1 tsp. vanilla
organic coconut oil

In a large bowl, mix together dry ingredients (flour, flaxseed meal, baking soda, baking powder, sea salt, cinnamon, cardamom, raisins, pecans). In a separate bowl, combine zucchini, agave nectar, soy milk, beaten eggs, and vanilla. Pour combined liquid ingredients into dry ingredient mixture. Stir by hand until ingredients are moistened. Grease medium-sized muffin pan with organic coconut oil. Fill each muffin well about $^3/_4$ full with muffin batter. Bake at 375°F for 15–20 minutes or until slightly browned. Allow to cool before eating. Stores well in freezer.

THANK-YOU RICE PAPER ROLLS

Infuse your rice with messages of thanks
About 4 rolls

1 package of rice paper wrappers
Several leaves of romaine or iceberg lettuce
1 cup white jasmine rice, cooked and cooled
1 cup cilantro, washed and chopped
$^1/_4$ cup cucumber, washed and cut into small cubes
$^1/_8$ cup carrots, shredded
1 cup bean sprouts
1 cup extra firm tofu, cubed
Crushed peanuts

Pour hot water into a shallow wide bowl that will fit the diameter of the rice paper wrapper. Gently take a rice paper wrapper from the package and place it into the bowl of warm water. Allow it to sit for a minute or until it becomes soft. Once soft, remove and place on a clean cutting board or large plate. Put lettuce leaf on top, and then add small amounts of rice, cilantro, cucumber, carrots, bean sprouts, tofu, and crushed peanuts. Roll up the wrap tightly and tuck in edges. Serve rolls plain or with a dipping sauce.

HEART-Y SPLIT PEA SOUP

Connects heart and solar plexus chakras, enabling love to empower you
Serves 6

1 Tbsp. extra-virgin olive oil
1 small yellow onion, diced
1 bay leaf
3 cloves garlic, peeled and minced
2 cups dried green split peas
1-$^1/_2$ tsp. sea salt
11 cups water
2 carrots, chopped
1 leek, chopped
3 celery stalks, chopped
$^1/_2$ cup parsley, chopped
$^1/_2$ tsp. dried basil
Dash fresh ground pepper

In a large pot over medium-high heat, sauté oil, onion, bay leaf, and garlic for 3–4 minutes or until onions are soft and translucent. Add the peas, salt, and water. Bring to boil and reduce heat to low. Simmer for 90 minutes, stirring occasionally. Add the carrots, leek, celery, parsley, basil, and ground pepper. Simmer for about 45 minutes, or until peas and vegetables are tender.

GREEN GARBANZO BEANS WITH LOVE RICE

Cultivates harmonious heart and solar plexus energies
Serves 4

5 cups water
1 cup dried green garbanzo beans
1-$^1/_2$ cups brown basmati rice
$^1/_2$ tsp. sea salt
$^1/_2$ cup walnuts
1 handful basil
2 cloves garlic
1 Tbsp. lemon juice

2 Tbsp. extra-virgin olive oil
$^1/_2$ cup celery, diced
Fresh ground pepper to taste

Bring water to boil and add beans, rice, and salt. Simmer, covered, for about 40 minutes. Remove from heat and let sit with cover on for about 10 minutes. Remove cover and allow to cool. While beans and rice are cooking, blend walnuts, basil, garlic, lemon juice, olive oil in a food processor. When beans and rice are cool, stir in nut-basil mixture and celery, and add pepper to taste.

SESAME KALE AND SPINACH TANGO

The king and queen of the greens to feed the heart chakra kingdom
Serves 2–3

1 bag fresh organic spinach, washed
1 bunch dinosaur kale, washed, chopped
1 green onion, chopped
2 cloves garlic, peeled and minced
1 tsp. sesame seeds
1 Tbsp. sesame oil

In a covered saucepan, cook spinach and kale on medium heat until wilted but still bright green. While greens are cooking, use separate pan to stir-fry green onion, garlic, and sesame seeds in sesame oil until sesame seeds are slightly browned. Add to drained, cooked greens, mix well, and serve either hot or chilled.

TO SUPPORT THE THROAT CHAKRA

SPICY NUT SAUCE

Sparks you to speak up
About 1 cup

$^1/_2$ cup organic crunchy peanut butter
$^1/_2$ cup organic cashew nut butter

4 Tbsp. black or green tea
1 tsp. sesame oil
2 Tbsp. soy sauce
1 Tbsp. rice vinegar
1 tsp. agave nectar
1 clove garlic, peeled and minced
$^1/_4$ tsp. crushed red pepper

Combine all ingredients. Spoon over steamed green vegetables or use as dipping sauce for rice or vegetable rolls.

MANGO CHUTNEY

A delicious delight!
About 4 cups

1 Tbsp. canola oil
1 tsp. cayenne pepper
1 Tbsp. curry powder
$^3/_4$ cup diced yellow onion
2 Tbsp. minced fresh ginger
$^1/_2$ cup diced orange bell pepper
$^1/_2$ cup golden raisins
3 cups fresh, ripe mangoes (roughly 2 mangoes), peeled and cut into strips
$^1/_2$ cup unsweetened pineapple juice
$^1/_2$ cup apple cider vinegar
1 cup agave nectar

In a small skillet, heat the oil and add the cayenne pepper, curry powder, and onion. Once onions become soft, add the ginger, raisins, and bell pepper and continue sautéing for 1 minute. Add the mango and cook for another minute. In a small mixing bowl, combine the pineapple juice, vinegar, and agave nectar. Add this mixture to the skillet. Simmer on low heat, stirring frequently, for 20–25 minutes, or until slightly thickened. Allow to cool, and pour into glass jar for storage.

BALSAMIC VINEGAR–PEACH SAUCE

Balances realms of the opposites
About $^1/_2$ cup

$^1/_2$ cup balsamic vinegar
$^1/_2$ cup fresh peaches, chopped
2 Tbsp. dried cranberries
1 Tbsp. walnut oil
1 Tbsp. walnuts, finely chopped

Simmer balsamic vinegar with peaches in a small skillet over medium heat until it turns to a syrup-like texture (about $1\text{-}^1/_2$ minutes). Remove from heat. Add dried cranberries, walnut oil, and walnuts. Drizzle on vegetables or chill and use as a salad dressing.

SEA PLANT VEGGIES

Encourages your authentic depths to surface
Serves 2

1 cup dulse, soaked and sliced into bite-sized bits
1 cup shredded carrots
1 cup alfalfa sprouts
3 red radishes, sliced
1 tsp. sesame oil
1 Tbsp. sesame seeds
Pinch sea salt

In mixing bowl, combine all ingredients. Serve cold.

VEGETARIAN NORI ROLLS

Spirals you back to your truth . . .
6 long nori rolls

2 cups cooked brown rice
2 Tbsp. rice vinegar
6 sheets pressed nori

Filling:

$^1/_4$ cup grated cucumber

$^1/_4$ cup alfalfa sprouts

$^1/_4$ cup purple cabbage

1 tsp. tamari or soy sauce

1 tsp. sesame seeds

Combine all ingredients for filling and set aside. Mix vinegar into rice. Place a single sheet of nori on a heavy cloth napkin to facilitate rolling. Spread $^1/_2$ cup rice over the sheet, leaving about a 1- to 2-inch edge. Put $^1/_4$ cup of filling down the middle on the flattened rice. Roll the nori. Eat as long nori stick, or cut to 1-inch pieces.

ASIAN MISO-DULSE SOUP

Gentle healing soup for the throat conduit
Serves 2–4

5 cups water

1-$^1/_2$ cups shredded bok choy and Chinese cabbage

3 large shiitake mushrooms, sliced

1 green onion, finely chopped

1 cup dulse

3 Tbsp. red miso

1 cup of extra-firm tofu, cubed

Sea salt, pinch

In a pot, add water, bok choy, cabbage, mushrooms, onion, dulse, and miso and allow to heat on low to medium heat for about 10 minutes. Add the tofu, and salt, if desired Serve immediately.

SEA-SLAW

Helps the throat chakra to balance
Serves 4–6

1 small red cabbage, grated or chopped

1 small green cabbage, grated or chopped

2 carrots, grated

1 cup dulse, soaked and sliced

2 Tbsp. orange juice

$^1/_2$ cup apple cider vinegar

1 Tbsp. caraway seeds

Sea salt and fresh ground pepper to taste

Combine ingredients and serve cold.

TO SUPPORT THE THIRD EYE CHAKRA

GREEN TEA—BERRY FREEZE

Allows you to awaken to your intuitive sight

Serves 2

1 cup water

2 green tea bags

2 cups frozen mixed berries (blueberries, raspberries, blackberries)

1-$^1/_2$ cups organic coconut (or soy) milk

$^1/_4$ cup pomegranate juice

Agave nectar to taste

Boil water and add to tea bags. Steep for 5 minutes. In meantime, combine mixed berries, milk, and juice in a blender until smooth. Add tea to berry blend and agave nectar for sweetness, if desired. Drink as a smoothie or freeze if you prefer to eat as a sorbet.

CHOCO-FFEE TOFU INSIGHT WHIP

Feeds your imagination

Serves 2–3

1 10-oz. package of firm tofu, drained

$^1/_2$ cup agave nectar

$^1/_4$ tsp. cinnamon

$^1/_4$ tsp. cardamom

1 tsp. instant coffee granules
1 tsp. shredded unsweetened coconut
2 Tbsp. cocoa
$^1/_2$ tsp. vanilla

Blend all ingredients until smooth. Place in a bowl, cover, and chill for 3–4 hours. Serve chilled.

CH-EYE TEA

Prepares you for the richness of your dream world
Serves 2–3

4 tsp. loose black (for example, Darjeeling) or green tea
1 cup water
$^1/_4$-inch ginger root, sliced thin
1 cinnamon stick, crushed
6 cardamom pods, crushed
3 cloves
2 cups cow's milk or soy milk
Agave nectar or stevia (optional)

In a saucepan, boil tea in 1 cup water. Allow to steep for 5 minutes. Add ginger, cinnamon, cardamom, cloves, and milk. Heat mixture on low to medium-high heat for 2 minutes, stirring occasionally. Remove from heat. Let sit for 2 minutes. Add agave nectar or stevia to sweeten. Serve warm.

BERRY WISDOM SEEKER COBBLER

Learn from the wisdom locked within berries
Serves 4–6

2 cups blueberries
1 cup blackberries
$^1/_4$ cup agave nectar
$^1/_4$ tsp. cinnamon
$^1/_4$ tsp. vanilla extract
1 cup organic rolled oats (not instant)

$^1/_4$ tsp. stevia
3 Tbsp. brown rice flour, sifted
1-$^1/_2$ Tbsp. organic butter, softened

Preheat oven to 350°F. Gently mix berries, agave nectar, cinnamon, and vanilla in a medium-sized bowl. Place in an 8-inch baking pan. In separate bowl, combine oats, stevia, brown rice flour, and butter. Mix with fingers until all ingredients are crumbly. Spoon on top of fruit mixture. Bake 35–40 minutes or until slightly browned. Cool before serving. Serve with organic vanilla yogurt.

GINGER SPICE BREAD

Rev up your third eye chakra with this tantalizing treat!
Serves 6–8

2 cups brown rice flour
1-$^1/_2$ tsp. baking soda
2 tsp. ground ginger
1 tsp. cardamom
1 tsp. cinnamon
1 tsp. nutmeg
$^1/_2$ tsp. sea salt
2 eggs
$^1/_2$ cup agave nectar
$^1/_2$ cup unsulphured molasses
2 Tbsp. fresh grated ginger
$^1/_2$ cup apple juice
$^1/_4$ cup canola or vegetable oil
1 tsp. orange zest

Preheat oven to 350°F. In a medium bowl, combine all dry ingredients: flour, baking soda, ground ginger, cardamom, cinnamon, nutmeg, sea salt. In a separate, large bowl, mix together eggs, agave nectar, molasses, fresh ginger, apple juice, oil, and orange zest. Slowly blend the dry mixture into the liquid ingredients so that they are evenly mixed. Pour into an 8-inch square baking pan. Bake for 30 minutes or until slightly browned. Cool before cutting and removing from pan. Cut into squares and serve.

TO SUPPORT THE CROWN CHAKRA

DETOX DYNAMO

Gives your crown chakra the strength to release stored toxins
Serves 1

Intention of "clarity"
1 organic apple (red or green), cored
1 organic carrot
1 organic celery stalk
$1/_2$-inch ginger root
$1/_2$ whole lemon
1 handful organic spinach leaves
Pinch cayenne pepper

With intention, juice all fruits and vegetables in a juicer. Add cayenne pepper, stir, and drink mindfully.

BERRY FLUSH

Flush stagnation from your crown with this colorful cleanse . . .
Serves 1

1 organic Red Delicious or Pink Lady apple, cored
1 cup organic strawberries, sliced
1 cup organic blueberries
$1/_2$ cup organic blackberries
Pinch cinnamon

Blend all ingredients in a blender or juicer. Infuse final mixture with "love" and "universal light and peace." Sip intentionally.

SUN-AND-FRUIT WATER

Makes it easy to stay hydrated and pure
About 1 gallon

1 gallon purified water
Sunny day
$^1/_2$ organic cucumber, sliced
2 slices organic orange
3 strawberries, sliced thinly, tops removed

Put water in a large glass pitcher in sunlight for 3–6 hours (10 ɒɪp ɪɪo
4 s ɪp ɪ). Add fruit. Gently stir. Pray that this water remove from your body
what needs clearing Sip throughout day.

GREEN GODDESS

Leverages the goodness of green to bring you back to God
Serves 1

1 organic cucumber
1 cup organic broccoli sprouts
1 stalk organic celery
1 organic green apple, cored
$^1/_8$ cup chopped mint
1 handful (organic) barley grass

Juice all ingredients in a juicer. Drink with intention to allow your body
and soul to connect fully with the Earth so that you can shed toxins from
your physical and spiritual layers.

DIVINE BROTH

A broth to sip during a cleaning fast
Serves 2

5 cups purified water
1 organic carrot, sliced
1 stalk organic celery, diced

$^1/_2$ cup parsley, chopped
1 organic green onion, finely sliced
$^1/_2$ cup chopped organic leeks
$^1/_4$ cup burdock root, chopped
1 Tbsp. fresh squeezed lemon juice
Sprinkle coarse sea salt

Boil water and add all ingredients listed. Gently simmer for 30 minutes. Serve warm.

SAMPLE CHAKRA-BALANCING MENUS

SAMPLE MENU #1*

Meal	Foods	Chakras Affected
Breakfast	Soy milk smoothie made with mango, hard-boiled egg, prayer of gratitude	Root, sacral, solar plexus, heart, throat, crown
Snack	Rye toast with almond butter, drizzled on top with agave nectar, black tea	Root, sacral, solar plexus, third eye
Lunch	Mixed green salad with cherry tomatoes, pine nuts, olives, carrots; plus I small cup lentil soup, small glass pomegranate juice, all infused with love	Root, sacral, solar plexus, heart, throat, crown
Snack	Plain, unsweetened yogurt with mixed berries and ground flaxseed meal	Root, sacral, heart, third eye
Dinner	Asian vegetable stir-fry (bamboo shoots, sprouts, snap peas, Chinese eggplant) with chicken, jasmine tea	Root, heart, throat, third eye
Snack	Baked apple with cinnamon	Root, third eye

*Note that regular eating times feed the solar plexus and throat chakras. Water to be sipped throughout the day feed the sacral chakra.

SAMPLE MENU #2

Meal	Foods	Chakras Affected
Breakfast	Steel-cut oatmeal with coconut milk, walnuts, agave nectar	Root, sacral, solar plexus
Snack	Iced tea made in sun, Bartlett pear, small handful of pecans	Root, sacral, heart, throat, third eye, crown
Lunch	Grilled tuna steak on bed of arugula with sesame oil dressing, passion fruit tea, meal shared with a friend	Root, sacral, heart, throat, third eye
Snack	Hummus with red pepper and carrots	Root, sacral, solar plexus
Dinner	Curried, cubed tofu with broccoli on basmati rice, cooked with gratitude	Root, solar plexus, heart, third eye
Snack	Mandarin orange	Sacral

SAMPLE MENU #3

Meal	Foods	Chakras Affected
Breakfast	Homemade high fiber, buckwheat/flax banana-walnut meal pancakes with blueberry compote	Root, sacral, solar plexus, heart, third eye
Snack	Chai tea with steamed soymilk, warm with blessings	Root, solar plexus, heart, third eye, crown
Lunch	Large sprouted whole grain tortilla filled with grilled vegetables (mushroom, zucchini, red peppers, eggplant, yellow summer squash), spinach, alfalfa sprouts, avocado slices, topped with tahini	Root, sacral, solar plexus, heart
Snack	Eat a peach using all your senses, intentionally sip roasted green tea	Sacral, heart, throat, third eye
Dinner	Homemade turkey chili with whole grain crackers, prayer of thanks	Root, solar plexus, crown
Snack	Trail mix (mixed nuts and fruits, unsweetened, shredded coconut)	Root, sacral, throat

APPENDIX A

List of Foods, Substances,
and Processes that Deplete the Chakras

Item	Root	Sacral	Solar Plexus	Heart	Throat	Third Eye	Crown
Artificial sweeteners	◆	◆	◆	◆	◆	◆	◆
Excessive alcohol	◆		◆			◆	
Excessive eating	◆		◆	◆	◆		◆
Excessive processed foods	◆	◆	◆	◆	◆	◆	◆
Excessive refined sugar			◆			◆	
Fast foods	◆	◆	◆	◆	◆		
Fried foods	◆	◆	◆	◆			
Genetically modified foods	◆						◆
High salt intake	◆	◆		◆	◆		
Mindless eating	◆				◆	◆	◆
Soft drinks	◆	◆	◆	◆	◆	◆	◆
Trans fats		◆		◆			◆
Use of pesticides	◆		◆				
Use of hormones and pharmaceuticals	◆	◆			◆	◆	

APPENDIX B

■ ■ ■ ■ ■ ■ ■ ■

List of Foods and Their Activating and Balancing Effects on the Chakras

✳   Activating

☉   Balancing

Item	Root	Sacral	Solar Plexus	Heart	Throat	Third Eye	Crown
FRUITS	✳☉	✳☉	✳☉	✳☉	✳☉	✳☉	
Apple, fresh, all	☉		☉				
Apple, dried			✳				
Apricot, fresh		☉					
Apricot, dried		✳					
Avocado		☉		☉			
Banana			✳				
Blackberries						☉	
Blood orange	✳	✳					
Blueberries						☉	
Boysenberries						☉	
Cantaloupe		☉			☉		
Coconut		☉					
Dates, dried			✳				
Dates, fresh			☉				
Elderberries						☉	
Fig		☉			☉		
Grapefruit	✳		✳				

Item	Root	Sacral	Solar Plexus	Heart	Throat	Third Eye	Crown
Grapes, green			⊙	⊙	⊙		
Grapes, purple			⊙		⊙	⊙	
Honeydew melon				⊙	⊙		
Kiwi		✸		✸	✸		
Kumquat		✸					
Lemon	✸		✸		✸		
Lime	✸				✸		
Mandarin orange		✸					
Mango		⊙			⊙		
Mango, dried		✸					
Marionberries						⊙	
Nectarine		⊙					
Orange		✸					
Papaya		⊙					
Passion fruit		⊙					
Peach		⊙			⊙		
Pear, green				⊙			
Pear, red	⊙						
Pineapple		✸	✸		✸		
Plantains			⊙				
Plum, dried (prune)			✸			✸	
Plum, red	⊙		⊙		⊙	⊙	
Plum, yellow			⊙		⊙		
Pomegranate	✸					⊙	
Raisins			✸			✸	
Raspberries	✸					⊙	
Red currants	✸					⊙	
Starfruit		✸	✸		✸		
Strawberries	✸						
Tangerine		✸					
Watermelon	⊙				⊙		

Item	Root	Sacral	Solar Plexus	Heart	Throat	Third Eye	Crown
NUTS	⊙	⊙				⊙	
Almonds	⊙	⊙					
Brazil nuts	⊙	⊙					
Cashews	⊙	⊙					
Filberts	⊙	⊙					
Hazelnuts	⊙	⊙					
Macadamia	⊙	⊙					
Pecans	⊙	⊙					
Pine nuts	⊙	⊙					
Pistachios	⊙	⊙					
Walnuts	⊙	⊙				⊙	
DAIRY	⊙	⊙					
Butter	⊙	⊙					
Buttermilk	⊙						
Cottage cheese	⊙						
Cream	⊙	⊙					
Eggs	⊙						
Feta cheese	⊙						
Ghee	⊙	⊙					
Kefir	⊙	⊙					
Milk, cow	⊙						
Milk, goat	⊙						
Milk, sheep	⊙						
Mozzarella	⊙						
Parmesan	⊙						
Yogurt, plain	⊙	⊙					
VEGETABLES	✳⊙	⊙	✳⊙	✳⊙	✳⊙	✳⊙	
Arame					⊙		
Artichoke			⊙	⊙			
Arugula				⊙			
Asparagus				⊙			

Item	Root	Sacral	Solar Plexus	Heart	Throat	Third Eye	Crown
Beet	⊙						
Bitter melon			✹	✹			
Bok choy				⊙			
Broccoflower				⊙			
Broccoli				⊙			
Brussels sprouts				⊙			
Cabbage, Chinese				⊙			
Cabbage, green				⊙			
Cabbage, red	⊙			⊙			
Cabbage, savoy				⊙			
Carrots	⊙	⊙	⊙				
Cauliflower				⊙			
Celery				⊙			
Chard, rainbow				⊙			
Chard, red	⊙			⊙			
Collard greens				⊙			
Corn			✹				
Cucumber				⊙	⊙		
Daikon	⊙			⊙			
Dandelion greens				⊙			
Dulse					⊙		
Eggplant			⊙			⊙	
Endive				⊙			
Garlic clove	✹		✹				
Gingerroot	✹		✹			✹	
Green peas			⊙	⊙			
Hijiki					⊙		
Horseradish				✹		✹	
Iceberg lettuce				⊙			
Kale, green				⊙			
Kale, purple				⊙		⊙	
Kelp					⊙		

Item	Root	Sacral	Solar Plexus	Heart	Throat	Third Eye	Crown
Leek	✹			☉			
Mesclun				☉			
Mushroom, button	☉						
Mushroom, chanterelle	☉						
Mushroom, crimini	☉						
Mushroom, enoki	☉						
Mushroom, maitake	☉						
Mushroom, morel	☉						
Mushroom, oyster	☉						
Mushroom, portobello	☉						
Mushroom, reishi	☉						
Mushroom, shiitake	☉						
Nori						☉	
Olives	☉	☉		☉			
Onions, green	✹		✹		✹		
Onions, red	✹		✹				
Onions, yellow	✹		✹				
Parsnip	☉		☉				
Peppers, green				☉	☉	☉	
Peppers, orange		☉	☉			☉	
Peppers, red	☉			☉		☉	
Peppers, yellow			☉			☉	
Potato, gold	☉		✹				
Potato, red	☉		✹				
Potato, sweet	☉	☉	☉				
Potato, white	☉		✹				
Pumpkin		☉	☉				
Radicchio				☉			
Radish	✹						
Romaine				☉			

Item	Root	Sacral	Solar Plexus	Heart	Throat	Third Eye	Crown
Rutabaga	⊙		⊙				
Sage				⊙			
Shallots	✹						
Spinach	⊙			⊙			
Sprouts, all				✹			
Squash, acorn	⊙		⊙				
Squash, winter	⊙		⊙				
Taro	⊙		⊙				
Tomato	✹					✹	
Turnip	⊙		⊙				
Wakame					⊙		
Wasabi	✹			✹			
Watercress				✹			
Yam	⊙	⊙	⊙				
Yucca	⊙		⊙				
Zucchini			⊙	⊙			
LEGUMES	⊙	⊙	⊙	⊙			
Adzuki beans	⊙		⊙				
Bean soup	⊙		⊙				
Black beans	⊙		⊙				
Black-eyed peas	⊙		⊙				
Butter beans			⊙				
Cannellini beans	⊙		⊙				
Fava beans	⊙		⊙				
Garbanzo beans (chickpea)	⊙		⊙				
Green beans	⊙		⊙	⊙			
Great Northern	⊙		⊙	⊙			
Hummus	⊙		⊙				
Kidney beans	⊙		⊙				
Lentils	⊙		⊙				
Lima beans			⊙				

Item	Root	Sacral	Solar Plexus	Heart	Throat	Third Eye	Crown
Miso		⊙		⊙			
Mung bean	⊙		⊙	⊙			
Navy beans	⊙		⊙				
Pinto	⊙		⊙				
Refried, fat-free	⊙		⊙				
Soy yogurt, unsweetened	⊙		⊙	⊙			
Soybean (edamame)	⊙		⊙				
Soy milk, unsweetened	⊙		⊙	⊙			
Tempeh	⊙	⊙	⊙	⊙			
Tofu	⊙		⊙	⊙			
GRAINS	⊙		✸⊙				
Amaranth			⊙				
Barley			⊙				
Buckwheat			⊙				
Bulgur (wheat)			⊙				
Cornmeal			✸				
Couscous (wheat)			⊙				
Millet			⊙				
Oat groats			⊙				
Quinoa	⊙		⊙				
Rice, basmati			⊙				
Rice, brown			⊙				
Rice, purple			⊙			⊙	
Rice, red	⊙		⊙			⊙	
Rice, white			✸⊙				
Rye			⊙				
Spelt			⊙				
Triticale			⊙				
Wheat			⊙				

Item	Root	Sacral	Solar Plexus	Heart	Throat	Third Eye	Crown
SWEETENERS	✸		✸⊙		✸	⊙	
Agave nectar			✸				
Brown rice syrup			✸				
Evaporated cane juice			✸				
Fructose			⊙				
Fruit juice concentrate			✸		✸		
High-fructose corn syrup			✸				
Honey			✸				
Maple syrup	✸		✸				
Molasses	✸		✸				
Powdered sugar			✸				
Raw sugar			✸				
Stevia			⊙			⊙	
MEAT	✸	⊙					
Beef	✸						
Buffalo	✸						
Chicken	✸						
Duck	✸	⊙					
Lamb	✸						
Ostrich	✸						
Pork	✸						
Turkey	✸						
Veal	✸						
Venison	✸						
SEAFOOD	✸⊙	⊙					
Anchovies	✸	⊙					
Catfish	⊙	⊙					
Cod	⊙	⊙					
Crab	⊙	⊙					
Haddock	⊙	⊙					
Halibut	⊙	⊙					
Herring	⊙	⊙					

Item	Root	Sacral	Solar Plexus	Heart	Throat	Third Eye	Crown
Lobster	☀	⊙					
Mackerel	⊙	⊙					
Menhaden	⊙	⊙					
Mussels	⊙	⊙					
Orange roughy	⊙	⊙					
Oyster	⊙	⊙					
Perch	⊙	⊙					
Red snapper	☀	⊙					
Rockfish	⊙	⊙					
Salmon	⊙	⊙					
Sardines	⊙	⊙					
Scrod	⊙	⊙					
Sea bass	⊙	⊙					
Sole	⊙	⊙					
Trout	⊙	⊙					
Whitefish	⊙	⊙					
OILS & NON-DAIRY FATS		⊙				⊙	
Almond oil		⊙				⊙	
Canola (rapeseed) oil		⊙					
Coconut milk		⊙					
Coconut oil		⊙					
Flaxseed oil		⊙				⊙	
Hemp oil		⊙				⊙	
Olive oil		⊙					
Peanut oil		⊙					
Pumpkin seed oil		⊙					
Rice bran oil		⊙					
Safflower oil		⊙					
Sunflower oil		⊙					
Walnut oil		⊙				⊙	

Item	Root	Sacral	Solar Plexus	Heart	Throat	Third Eye	Crown
SEEDS	⊙	⊙	⊙			✻⊙	
Flax		⊙	⊙			⊙	
Hemp		⊙				✻	
Poppy		⊙				✻	
Psyllium		⊙	⊙				
Pumpkin	⊙	⊙					
Sesame	⊙	⊙	⊙			⊙	
Sunflower	⊙	⊙	⊙				
Tahini	⊙	⊙	⊙			⊙	
BEVERAGES	✻⊙	✻⊙	✻		⊙	✻⊙	⊙
Coffee						✻	
Juice, apple	⊙		✻		⊙		
Juice, grape			✻		⊙	✻	
Juice, grapefruit		✻	✻		⊙		
Juice, orange		✻	✻		⊙		
Juice, pineapple		✻	✻		⊙		
Juice, tomato	⊙		✻		⊙		
Tea, black					⊙	✻	
Tea, green				✻	⊙	✻	
Tea, herbal		⊙			⊙	⊙	
Water		⊙			⊙		⊙
Wine, red	✻					✻	
Wine, white						✻	
SPICES	✻	✻	✻	✻		✻	
Allspice						✻	
Anise						✻	
Basil				✻		✻	
Bay leaf				✻		✻	
Black pepper	✻		✻			✻	
Caraway		✻				✻	
Cardamom			✻			✻	
Cayenne	✻		✻			✻	
Chili powder	✻					✻	
Chives				✻		✻	

Item	Root	Sacral	Solar Plexus	Heart	Throat	Third Eye	Crown
Cinnamon			✳			✳	
Cloves	✳					✳	
Coriander			✳			✳	
Cumin	✳		✳			✳	
Curry			✳			✳	
Dill				✳		✳	
Fennel		✳		✳		✳	
Fenugreek			✳			✳	
Ginger	✳		✳			✳	
Horseradish	✳		✳	✳		✳	
Lemon verbena			✳			✳	
Majoram				✳		✳	
Mint				✳		✳	
Nutmeg	✳	✳	✳			✳	
Oregano				✳		✳	
Paprika	✳					✳	
Parsley				✳		✳	
Rosemary				✳		✳	
Sage				✳		✳	
Tarragon				✳		✳	
Thyme				✳		✳	
Turmeric	✳		✳			✳	
Wasabi	✳		✳	✳		✳	
MISCELLANEOUS	✳☾	✳⊙	✳⊙	✳⊙	⊙	✳⊙	⊙
Chocolate, dark						✳	
Chocolate, milk	✳		✳			✳	
Vinegar			✳			✳	
Organically grown	☾			⊙			⊙
Prepared with love	☾	⊙	⊙	⊙	⊙	⊙	⊙
Non-GMO	☾						⊙
Wild, free-range animals	☾	⊙	⊙	⊙	⊙	⊙	⊙

APPENDIX C

Chakras and Corresponding Foods

Chakra	Symbol	Qualities	Food/Drink to Activate	Food/Drink to Balance
Root	■	Grounding Protective Earthy	Meat, acidic fruits and vegetables, garlic, ginger, spicy root vegetables, dense and dark sweeteners, red seafood, select spices	Specific fruits, nuts, dairy products, red vegetables, root vegetables, mushrooms, legumes, specific grains, most seafood, seeds, certain juices
Sacral	●	Creative Flowing Sensual	Dried orange fruits, acidic fruits, select fruit juices, and spices	Orange fruits and vegetables, melons, fruits high in fat, tropical fruits, nuts, high-fat dairy, plant-based oils, seafood, seeds, water, duck
Solar Plexus	▲	Energetic Powerful Fiery	Dried fruits, yellow fruits, acidic fruits, ginger, potatoes, corn, white rice, most sweeteners, most juices, some spices, vinegar	Select fruits, certain yellow fruits, pine nuts, select vegetables, certain legumes, most whole grains, fructose, psyllium

Chakras	Symbol	Qualities	Food/Drink to Activate	Food/Drink to Balance
Heart	◆	Compassionate Loving Joyful	Bitter melon, spicy (green) vegetables (for example, horseradish, wasabi), spices from green plants	Nonacidic green fruits, green vegetables, cruciferous vegetables, chlorophyll, certain legumes, soy products
Throat	★	Truthful Communicative Synchronizing	Select sour fruits, tomatoes, fruit juice concentrate	Melons, figs, plums, watermelon, cucumbers, sea plants, bell peppers, fruit juice
Third Eye	◎	Intuitive Insightful Intense	Wine, spices, coffee, chocolate	Berries, red/purple fruits, vegetables and grains, walnuts, almonds, stevia, certain oils, sesame products
Crown	☀	Pure Clarifying Divine	Prayer	Purified water, sunlight, clean air

Health Conditions and Corresponding Chakras*

Health Condition	Root	Sacral	Solar Plexus	Heart	Throat	Third Eye	Crown
Acne	●						
Addictions	○	●	●	●	●	●	
Adrenal fatigue	○		⊙			●	
Alcoholism	○		⊙			●	
Allergies	○		⊙		●		
Alzheimer's disease						⊙	●
Anemia	○			●			
Anorexia	○				●	●	●
Anxiety	●		●	⊙	●	●	●
Asthma				●	⊙		
Atherosclerosis (thickening of arteries)				●			
Attention deficit disorder (ADD)			●			⊙	
Autoimmune disease	○						●
Back pain, low	○	●					
Back pain, middle			⊙	●			
Back pain, upper				●	⊙		
Bladder infection (men)		●					
(women)		●					

---

*Chakra most connected to that condition indicated by a ⊙

Health Condition	Root	Sacral	Solar Plexus	Heart	Throat	Third Eye	Crown
Bloating		☉	✳				
Blood pressure, high	✳			☉			
Blood pressure, low	✳			☉			
Bone fracture	✳						
Breast problems (cysts, lumps, soreness)		✳		☉			
Breathing difficulty				✳	☉		
Bronchitis				☉	✳		
Bruises	✳			✳			
Bulimia	✳		☉		✳	✳	
Cancer		✳					
Candida overgrowth		✳					
Carpal tunnel syndrome				☉			✳
Cataracts						✳	
Celiac disease		☉	✳				
Colds (upper respiratory)	☉			✳	✳		
Colitis	✳	☉					
Constipation	✳	☉					
Coughing				✳	☉		
Crohn's disease	☉	✳					
Cystitis	✳	☉					
Depression	✳					✳	☉
Diabetes			✳				
Diarrhea	✳	☉					
Ear infection	✳				☉		
Excessive appetite	✳	✳	☉		✳	✳	
Farsightedness						✳	
Fatigue	✳		☉			✳	
Fever	✳						

Health Condition	Root	Sacral	Solar Plexus	Heart	Throat	Third Eye	Crown
Flatulence (gas)	✸	✸	⊙		✸		
Flu	○	✸	✸		✸	✸	
Gallstones			✸				
Gastritis			✸				
Goiter					✸		
Gout	✸						
Gum disease	✸			✸	⊙		
Hair loss	○						✸
Halitosis (bad breath)					✸		
Hay fever	⊙				✸		
Headaches						⊙	✸
Hearing loss					✸		
Heart attack				✸			
Heartburn			✸				
Hemorrhoids	✸						
Herpes	✸	✸					
High blood sugar (hyperglycemia)			✸				
High cholesterol				✸			
Hives	✸						
Hyperactivity			✸			⊙	
Hyperthyroidism			✸		⊙		
Hypothyroidism	✸		✸		⊙		
Impotence	✸						
Incontinence	✸	⊙					
Indigestion		✸	⊙	✸	✸		
Inflammation	✸						
Insomnia						✸	
Itching	⊙						✸
Jaw tightness (TMJ)					✸		

Health Condition	Root	Sacral	Solar Plexus	Heart	Throat	Third Eye	Crown
Kidney stones	✸	⊙					
Knee pain	✸						
Laryngitis					✸		
Left side of body complaints		⊙		✸		✸	
Leukemia	⊙	✸					
Liver problems (hepatitis, jaundice)			✸				
Low blood sugar (hypoglycemia)			✸				
Lupus	⊙						✸
Menstrual problems		✸					
Migraines						✸	
Motion sickness					⊙	✸	
Multiple sclerosis	⊙						✸
Nausea			✸		⊙		
Nearsightedness						✸	
Neck pain					✸		
Nerve pain	✸						⊙
Numbness							⊙
Obesity	⊙		✸		✸		
Osteoarthritis	✸						
Osteoporosis	✸						
Parasites	✸						
Pneumonia	✸			⊙	✸		
Poor circulation	⊙			✸			
Premenstrual syndrome		✸					
Prostate problems	✸						
Psoriasis	✸						
Rash	✸						
Rheumatoid arthritis	✸						
Right side of body complaints	⊙		✸		✸		

Health Condition	Root	Sacral	Solar Plexus	Heart	Throat	Third Eye	Crown
Runny or stuffy nose	✹				⊙		
Schizophrenia						✹	
Sciatica	✹						⊙
Seizures						⊙	✹
Senility						⊙	✹
Sinus congestion	✹				⊙		
Snoring			✹		✹		
Stomach ulcers			✹				
Stroke	✹			⊙		✹	✹
Stuttering					⊙		
Sty						✹	
Swelling (edema)		✹					
Tooth pain or problems	✹				⊙		
Urinary tract infection	✹	⊙					
Vaginitis	✹	⊙					
Varicose veins	⊙			✹			
Venereal disease	✹	⊙					
Yeast infections	✹	⊙					

BIBLIOGRAPHY

Chapter 1
Emoto, Masaru. *The True Power of Water: Healing and Discovering Ourselves.* Beyond Words Publishing, 2005.

Chapter 2
Gerber, Richard. *Vibrational Medicine: New Choices for Healing Ourselves.* Bear & Co., 1996.

Chapter 4
Colbin, Annemarie. *Food and Healing.* Ballantine Books, 1986.

Chapter 5
McCraty, R., M. Atkinson, W.A. Tiller, G. Rein, and A.D. Watkins. "The effects of emotions on short-term power spectrum analysis of heart rate variability." *Am J Cardiol.* 1995 Nov 15;76(14): 1089–93.

Owen, Harrison. *The Power of Spirit: How Organizations Transform.* Berrett-Koehler Publishers, 2000.

Sternini, C., L. Anselmi and E. Rozengurt. "Enteroendocrine Cells. A Site of 'Taste' in Gastrointestinal Chemosensing." *Curr Opin Endocrinol Diabetes Obes.* 2008 Feb; 15(1): 73–8.

Chapter 6
Arrien, Angeles. *The Four-Fold Way: Walking the Paths of the Warrior, Teacher, Healer, and Visionary.* Harper One, 1993.

Myss, Caroline. *Anatomy of the Spirit: The Seven Stages of Power and Healing.* Three Rivers Press, 1997.

Chapter 7

Christakis, N. A., and J. H. Fowler. "The spread of obesity in a large social network over 32 years." *N Engl J Med.* 2007;357(4): 370–79.

Dossey, Larry. "Compassion." *Explore* 2007; 3(1): 1–5.

Gerrard, Don. *One Bowl: A Guide to Eating for Body and Spirit.* Da Capo Press, 2001.

McCraty, Rollin. *The Energetic Heart: Bioelectromagnetic Interactions within and between People.* Institute of HeartMath, 2003.

Walsh, M. C., L. Brennan, E. Pujos-Guillot, J. L. Sébédio, A. Scalbert, A. Fagan, D. G. Higgins, and M. J. Gibney. "Influence of acute phytochemical intake on human urinary metabolomic profiles." *Am J Clin Nutr.* 2007; 86(6): 1687–93.

Chapter 8

Hoch, S. J., E. L. Bradlow, and B. Wansink. "The variety of assortment." *Marketing Science* 1999; 18(4): 527-46.

Kahn, B. E. and B. Wansink. "The influence of assortment structure on perceived variety and consumption quantities." *Journal of Consumer Research* 2004; 30(4): 519–33.

Chapter 9

Macdiarmid, J. I., and M. M. Hetherington. "Mood modulation by food: an exploration of affect and cravings in 'chocolate addicts.'" *Br J Clin Psychol.* 1995; 34 (Pt 1): 129-38.

Michener, W., and P. Rozin. "Pharmacological versus sensory factors in the satiation of chocolate craving." *Physiol Behav.* 1994; 56(3): 419–22.

Chapter 10

Gerrard, Don. *One Bowl: A Guide to Eating for Body and Spirit.* Da Capo Press, 2001.

Myss, Caroline. *Anatomy of the Spirit: The Seven Stages of Power and Healing.* Three Rivers Press, 1997.

Jung, L. Shannon. *Food for Life: The Spirituality and Ethics of Eating.* Fortress Press, 2004.

INDEX

ABOUT THE AUTHOR

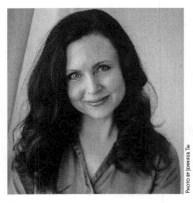

Deanna M. Minich, Ph.D., C.N., is an internationally known nutritionist, educator, researcher, counselor, and writer with more than fifteen years experience in the nutrition field, ranging from innovating products in the food and dietary supplement industries to counseling patients in private practice. Her traditional academic study of nutrition has merged with her study of ancient spiritual traditions like Reiki, yoga, the chakra system, and Shamanism to create the novel, integrated approach to food and eating presented in *Chakra Foods for Optimum Health*. Currently, Dr. Minich lives in Port Orchard, Washington, where she writes and teaches others about food and spirituality.

For More Information

Visit *www.foodandspirit.com* or contact Dr. Minich at deannaminich@hotmail.com.

TO OUR READERS

Conari Press, an imprint of Red Wheel/Weiser, publishes books on topics ranging from spirituality, personal growth, and relationships to women's issues, parenting, and social issues. Our mission is to publish quality books that will make a difference in people's lives—how we feel about ourselves and how we relate to one another. We value integrity, compassion, and receptivity, both in the books we publish and in the way we do business.

Our readers are our most important resource, and we value your input, suggestions, and ideas about what you would like to see published. Please feel free to contact us, to request our latest book catalog, or to be added to our mailing list.

Conari Press
An imprint of Red Wheel/Weiser, or
500 Third Street, Suite 230
San Francisco, CA 94107
www.redwheelweiser.com